Nick Vandome

iPhone & Apple Watch

for

Health & Fitness

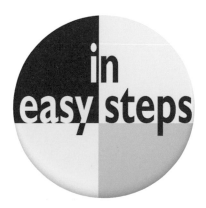

in
easy steps

In easy steps is an imprint of In Easy Steps Limited
16 Hamilton Terrace · Holly Walk · Leamington Spa
Warwickshire · United Kingdom · CV32 4LY
www.ineasysteps.com

Notice of Liability
Every effort has been made to ensure that this book contains accurate
and current information. However, In Easy Steps Limited and the
author shall not be liable for any loss or damage suffered by readers
as a result of any information contained herein.

Trademarks
iPhone® and Apple Watch® are registered trademarks of Apple
Computer, Inc. All other trademarks are acknowledged as belonging
to their respective companies.

In Easy Steps Limited supports The Forest Stewardship Council (FSC),
the leading international forest certification organization. All our titles
that are printed on Greenpeace approved FSC certified paper carry the
FSC logo.

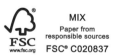

MIX
Paper from
responsible sources
FSC® C020837

Printed and bound in the United Kingdom

ISBN 978-1-84078-735-1

Contents

Preface

It is easy to get overwhelmed at the thought of improving health and fitness, but with the development of health and fitness devices and apps to support your endeavors, there has never been a better time to start a new regime that can help transform your life.

My own personal view of improving health and fitness is that it should be looked at as a long-term lifestyle goal, rather than a quick-fix for short-term gains (which may disappear as quickly as they are achieved). For instance, aiming to do 10% more exercise over the course of a year is an attainable goal without seeming too daunting or time-consuming. Once this has been done, incremental increases can be made so that, ideally, health and fitness becomes an embedded part of your life and not something that is seen as a chore or an obstacle.

Leading the sedentary life of a writer, I am conscious of the need to build health and fitness into my daily routine, whether this is going for a walk at lunchtime, or playing tennis and squash at every opportunity (team or club sports also have the added benefit of providing an active social circle). Using the devices and apps in this book has provided a genuine and significant help in recording health and fitness activities and also, by using them on a daily basis, has helped to keep me motivated to meet the goals that are set on the apps. Having said that, there are no devices or apps that can make you lace up your running shoes or put on your gym gear: ultimately, motivation and willpower for improving health and fitness has to come from your own determination and desire. Hopefully, **iPhone & Apple Watch for Health & Fitness in easy steps** will provide help, support and encouragement in creating, measuring and achieving your health and fitness goals.

Nick Vandome

1 Getting Healthy with Apple

Health and fitness is an area that fits perfectly with the iPhone and the Apple Watch. This chapter shows how they can be used for this, and some of the health apps to use.

The Health Revolution

It is hard to pinpoint when the idea of health and fitness became an industry rather than people's individual hobbies, but one legitimate claimant could be 1977 when the book *The Complete Book of Running* by Jim Fixx was published. This kickstarted the jogging craze in America, which not only promoted jogging and running as a form of exercise, but also extolled the health benefits that could be gained from it.

In the decades that followed the publication of *The Complete Book of Running*, health and fitness has become entrenched in the daily lives of millions of people: from enthusiasts undertaking events such as fun runs to full marathons, to cyclists joining their local clubs, and the thousands of health clubs and gyms that have opened to cater for this expanding industry. In addition, there has also been a raised general awareness of health and fitness issues, whether it is trying to walk a certain number of steps a day, or eating more fruit and vegetables.

Technology, Apple and health

Whenever there is a new and expanding industry, technology is never far away, providing gadgets and services to help motivate people and maintain their goals and targets. For health and fitness, this is done through a range of items, such as wearable devices for monitoring and recording activities, and an expanding number of apps covering topics from walking to yoga.

Apple is at the forefront of the partnership between technology and health; it has a number of options in this field and they are starting to be linked together so that information from one area can be shared with others. These include:

- **iPhone**. The iPhone has evolved into a device that can be used to record and monitor health and fitness data. It contains several motion and fitness sensors that can record body motion, steps walked and flights of steps climbed. It also has the Health app for recording a range of health data.

- **Health apps**. The App Store has a category for Health & Fitness apps that can be downloaded onto the iPhone.

- **Apple Watch**. First released in 2015, the Apple Watch is a wearable device that can be used to record workouts and activity through its apps and range of body sensors.

Don't forget

Health apps can also be downloaded onto the Apple Watch (via the iPhone) from the Apple App Store.

Don't forget

Apple Watch Series 2 was released in September 2016. In most respects is it similar to Series 1, except that it has GPS, is waterproof and has a higher specification processor and a brighter screen.

iPhone

The iPhone has a built-in Health app that can be used to record information about a range of items, from Fitness to Nutrition. Some of these are recorded automatically by the motion and fitness sensors, and some have to be entered manually. The motion and fitness sensors can also be used with third-party apps that have been downloaded from the App Store.

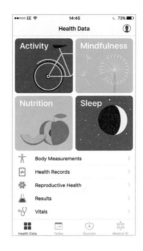

Health apps

The App Store has an expanding range of health and fitness apps, as the hardware that they use is able to track a wider range of functions. Apps cover general fitness activities such as running and cycling, workouts, and health and wellbeing activities such as yoga, Pilates and meditation.

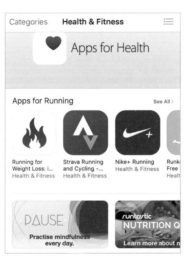

For a detailed look at using health and fitness apps from the App Store, see Chapter Three.

Apple Watch

The Apple Watch works in conjunction with the iPhone. On the back of the Apple Watch are sensors that can record readings such as body movement and heart rate. It has two main apps for recording health and fitness: the Activity app and the Workout app. Once information has been recorded, it can be sent to the iPhone for viewing and analysis.

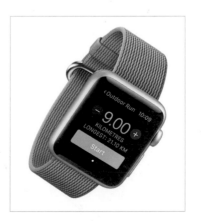

For a detailed look at using the Apple Watch, see Chapters Five-Six.

iPhone for Health

In addition to the Health app, the iPhone also has sensors that can monitor your movement. This can then be translated into information for the Health app, such as number of steps walked, or the number of flights of stairs climbed. The motion sensors can also be used with appropriate third-party apps. To do this:

In the Settings app, buttons that are **On** are colored green.

10

A lot of third party apps that use the Motion & Fitness sensors are step-counters (pedometers).

1   Access **Settings > Privacy** on your iPhone

2   Tap on the **Motion & Fitness** button

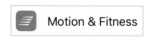

3   Drag the **Fitness Tracking** button to **On** to enable apps to use the Motion & Fitness sensors on the iPhone

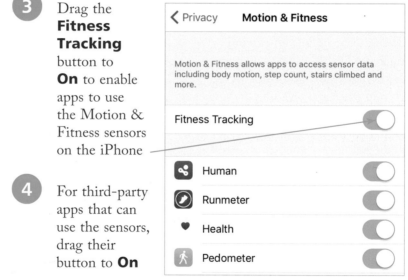

4   For third-party apps that can use the sensors, drag their button to **On**

5   Within the **Settings** app, third party apps can also be given access to the Motion & Fitness sensors. Access the app in the **Settings** app and drag the **Motion & Fitness** button to **On**

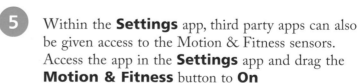

Apple Watch for Health

The latest version of the Apple Watch (at the time of printing) is the Apple Watch Series 2. This is the same in most regards as the Apple Watch Series 1, except that it is more waterproof, has an improved sensor and screen and has its own built-in GPS for tracking walking, running or cycling routes. The main health and fitness elements of the Apple Watch are:

Activity app
This can be used to measure your daily activity. It includes the amount of movement you do, the amount of exercise, and also the frequency which you stand during the day. It consists of three rings, which show your progress during the day towards your daily targets.

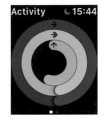

Workout app
This can be used to track your workout activities. Different workout options can be selected, e.g. walk, run, cycle, rowing machine or stair stepper, and criteria can then be set for each item. This can include setting the number of active calories you want to burn, distance or duration.

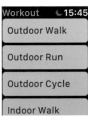

Breathe app
This is an app for relaxation and can be used to spend as little as a minute (or longer, as required) concentrating on inhaling and exhaling to provide a peaceful break to the stresses and strains of the day. It records each session so you can see how many times you have done this in a day, along with your heart rate while doing it.

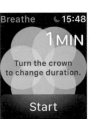

Heart Rate app
This can be used to display your current heart rate. This is done via the sensors on the bottom of the Apple Watch. The watch has to be connected to your wrist in order for a correct heart rate reading to be made.

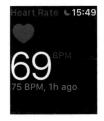

Integration with the Health app
The Apple Watch also works well with the Health app on the iPhone, and the two devices can share information via this app.

The functionality of the Apple Watch Series 1 and Series 2 is the same, and they both use the same operating system: WatchOS 3.

The Activity, Workout, Breathe and Heart Rate apps can work independently on the Apple Watch, but in order to share data from these apps, the iPhone and the Apple Watch have to be 'paired'.
See page 88 for details about pairing the Apple Watch and iPhone.

Monitoring Activity

Health and fitness apps on the iPhone monitor and display information in different ways, but there is a general consistency in the type of details displayed:

For a more detailed look at the Health app, see Chapter Two.

1 The **Health** app has sections for each topic, and the information is displayed on a colored graph

2 Topics can also be selected to appear on the Health app's **Today** page so that you can view a range of items on one screen

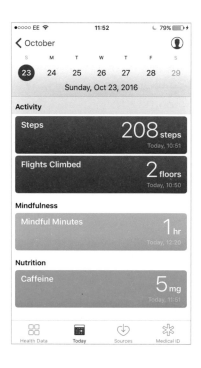

3 GPS apps track your route for activities such as walking, running or cycling, and show it on a map

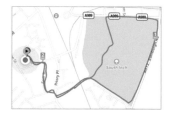

For a more detailed look at apps for walking and running (and cycling), see Chapter Four.

4 Step-counter and pedometer apps display information including numbers of steps taken, distance traveled and calories burned

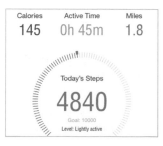

12

Health Apps

Most forms of healthy living and exercise are catered for with apps in the App Store, which can be downloaded to an iPhone and, in some cases, an Apple Watch. These can be found in the dedicated Health & Fitness category in the App Store. Some of the types of apps include:

Running and walking
These apps can be used to track the number of steps that you take when exercising, and also map your routes using GPS technology.

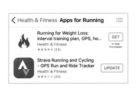

Fitness classes
These apps can be used to find fitness classes in your local area. Location Services has to be turned **On** in order for these to work properly.

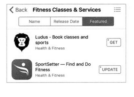

Timers
These apps can be used to time parts, or the whole, of workout routines. Different items can be timed and then compared when you do the same thing again.

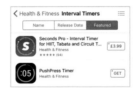

Workout routines
These apps contain quick workout routines that have animated images, and videos that can be followed.

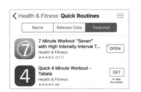

Healthy habits
These apps cover a range of healthy lifestyle areas, such as healthy eating, stopping smoking, calorie counters and combating stress and anxiety.

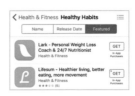

Meditation & mindfulness
These apps cover relaxation techniques such as yoga, Pilates, meditation, breathing exercises and calming sounds to aid sleep.

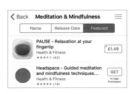

Running and walking apps using GPS can also be used for cycling.

Location Services can be found on the iPhone at **Settings** > **Privacy** > **Location Services** and drag **Location Services** to **On**.

Creating Healthy Routines

While technology and apps can help to motivate people with health and fitness, and store and analyze data, there is no substitute for personal motivation and willpower. Improving health and fitness should be viewed as a long-term change of lifestyle, rather than something for short-term gain that is going to be stopped once a certain target is achieved. As well as using the iPhone, Apple Watch and health apps, there are some areas that could be considered for a healthier and fitter lifestyle:

- **Create realistic goals**. One of the greatest ways to become demotivated when undertaking a new health and fitness regime is to fail to achieve any goals that you have set yourself. Therefore, it is important to set realistic goals that you think you can achieve, or surpass, so that you keep motivated. If you achieve your goals, consolidate this and then set new, equally realistic ones.

- **Do not expect an overnight transformation**. As well as being realistic, it is important not to expect too much in a short period of time: in fact, in some ways it is better not to put a timeframe on it at all. No-one will become an international athlete overnight, and the aim should be to change your lifestyle first and then benefits will accrue from this naturally.

- **Embed health and fitness in your daily routine**. Instead of making health and fitness feel like a chore that has to be fitted into the day, make it part of your daily routine. For instance, schedule a walk at lunchtime twice a week, and put this in your calendar so that there is a tangible reminder.

- **Keep a health and fitness notebook**. If you write down your health and fitness activities, this provides tangible evidence of what you have done. This can be used to motivate yourself by looking back at what you have already achieved, and also be used as a guide to build on and improve this.

- **Connect with like-minded people**. One of the best ways to keep motivated and enthused about health and fitness is to join with other people doing the same. This could mean joining a local club, or linking with other people doing the same things via social media such as Facebook and Twitter. This way, you can also provide encouragement for each other, which is one of the best ways to stay motivated.

See Chapter 10 for more information about maintaining a healthy lifestyle.

Keep a digital notebook of your activities on a note-taking app on the iPhone, such as the built-in Notes app.

Collating Health Data

When performing health and fitness activities, it is useful to be able to view data from these activities so that you can compare your progress with earlier periods. The data could be written down by hand, or added to a spreadsheet, but this can be laborious and liable to mistakes or missed entries. A more effective option is to use an app that can automatically record and display fitness information. The Apple Watch and iPhone offer one such app; the Activity app. The Apple Watch version can record the data, and display daily totals, while the iPhone version stores an archive of all of your activity and also displays a more in-depth record:

The three goals for the Activity app are: **Move** (which measures active calories, which are calories burned over your normal resting level); **Exercise** (which measures any activity over the level of a brisk walk; and **Stand** (which measures the number of hours during which you stand and move around for at least one minute).

1 The **Activity** app on the Apple Watch displays the progress towards meeting three daily goals, in ring format and with specific details

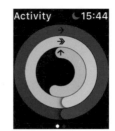

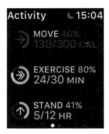

2 The **Activity** app on the iPhone displays the same information (within the **History** section) but with more detailed graphs, and calendar options at the top of the window for viewing activity data from other dates. Swipe to the left on a panel to view textual details of the data

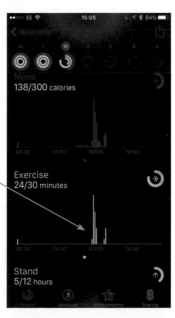

The History section also displays any awards that you have received for that day's activity, number of steps walked and distance covered. Swipe down the window to view these details.

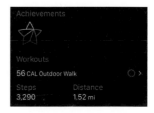

...cont'd

3 The **Activity** app also displays details from the Workout app, so all of your health and fitness activities can be viewed from the same app. Tap on a workout to view its details

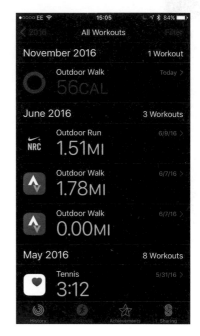

The thumbnails on the calendar in Step 4 display how much of the activities were completed for any given day.

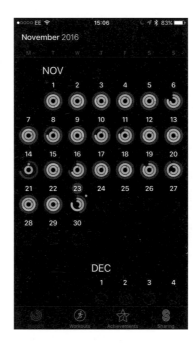

4 Tap on the month at the top of the screen in Step 2 to access the Activity app calendar. Tap on a date to view the relevant activity data

5 Data from the Activity app is also displayed in a panel in the Health app on the iPhone

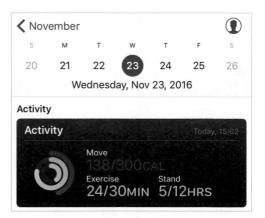

2 iPhone Health App

This Health app on the iPhone is a versatile app that can automatically record some health and fitness data and also display details from other apps. This chapter shows how to use the Health app for monitoring your health and fitness.

About the Health App

The Health app is a built-in app that comes with the operating system (iOS) on the iPhone. Tap on this icon to open the Health app:

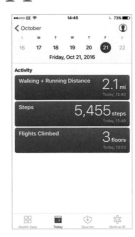

Tap on the bottom toolbar to access the sections within it.

The Health app is the starting point for displaying information about a range of health and fitness activities, including:

- General activity such as walking and running

- Nutrition

- Sleep

- Heart rate and blood pressure

- Medical data such as blood glucose and inhaler usage

Each category can have data added manually, while some categories, such as number of steps, can be updated automatically by the Health app and your iPhone.

The full range of categories in the Health app are accessed from the **Health Data** button on the bottom toolbar.

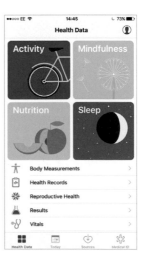

18

Apps with the Health app

Several of the categories within the Health app work in conjunction with third-party apps, which can be downloaded from the App Store. The apps can monitor the required function, and the data can be collated and displayed by the Health app. This can be used for any category where the Health app does not have the functionality for recording the required data. For instance, you could download an app to monitor your sleeping patterns, and collate the information in the Health app so that you can view it over a period of time (see pages 20-21 for details).

Adding your own data

When you are creating a picture of your health over a period of time, it is important to be able to enter information manually, for times when it cannot be done through your iPhone – e.g. if you do not have your iPhone with you, but you still want to include the number of steps from when you are walking. This can be done with the Add option for any category. Tap on the **+** button and then enter the details for the appropriate item (data points) and tap on the **Add** button.

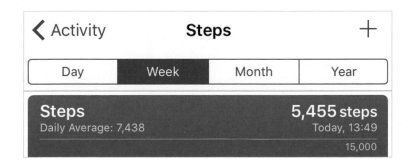

Data points can be added several times within the same day.

Data points can be deleted but their numerical values cannot be changed.

Accessories with the Health app

The Health app can display data for a range of medical vital statistics, through the use of third-party apps. However, for some of these, accessories are required in order for the app to function to its full potential. For instance, if you want to check your blood pressure with an appropriate app, you will also need a wireless blood pressure monitor. Once the information is recorded, it can be displayed within the Health app.

It is best to seek professional medical advice before using medical accessories with the Health app.

Using Third-Party Apps

The Health app can interact with a large number of third-party apps, so that they can display their data within the Health app. This means that the Health app can be used to view a range of data from numerous sources, rather than having to open each app separately. To use third-party apps with the Health app:

1 Within each Health app category there are suggested apps specific to the topic. Tap on one of the apps to download it directly from the App Store

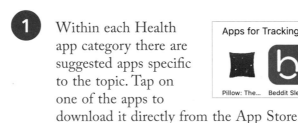

Apps for Tracking Sleep Analysis

Pillow: The...   Beddit Sle...   Sleep Cycl...   S+ by Res...

Third-party health and fitness apps do not have to be connected to the Health app, but if they are not, their data will not be available in the Health app.

2 Open the app. It will ask to connect to the Health app in order to share its data. Tap on the **Connect** button

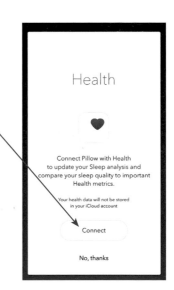

Health

Connect Pillow with Health to update your Sleep analysis and compare your sleep quality to important Health metrics.

Your health data will not be stored in your iCloud account

Connect

No, thanks

Two of the options in Step 3 are for the app to **Write** and **Read** data. If both options are **On**, this enables two-way communication between the third-party app and the Health app.

3 Tap **On** the required settings for the app, and then tap on the **Allow** button

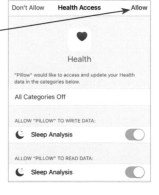

Don't Allow   **Health Access**   Allow

Health

"Pillow" would like to access and update your Health data in the categories below.

All Categories Off

ALLOW "PILLOW" TO WRITE DATA:

☾ Sleep Analysis

ALLOW "PILLOW" TO READ DATA:

☾ Sleep Analysis

4 Within the Health app, access a topic and tap on the **Data Sources & Access** button

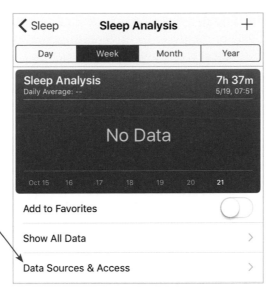

Within each topic, the panel at the top of the window shows all of the information that has been collated by the Health app, displayed by Day, Week, Month or Year.

5 Under the **Data Sources & Access** heading, drag this button to **On** to allow the Health app and the selected apps to communicate with each other

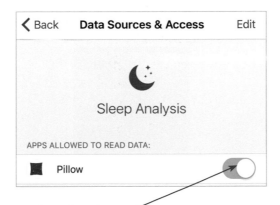

6 Once a third-party app has been connected to the Health app, its data is shown in the **All Recorded Data** section (accessed from the **Show All Data** button)

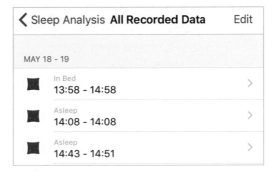

Health App Categories

The Health app covers a wide range of categories and topics. Some of these can be used on their own with data from the iPhone, such as Fitness; others, such as Body Measurements or Vitals, require information to be added manually. The current categories that are available in the Health app are all accessed from the Health Data button:

1 Tap on the **Health Data** button on the bottom toolbar to view all of the categories

Health Data

2 The main headings (**Activity**, **Mindfulness**, **Nutrition** and **Sleep**) are displayed at the top of the window. The other categories are listed below

Beware

Some of the categories and topics within the Health app have been developed with a view to being used with the Apple Watch, once it has all of the appropriate sensors to read the data.

Don't forget

Each category has its own default color, which is displayed when data from the category is used within the Health app.

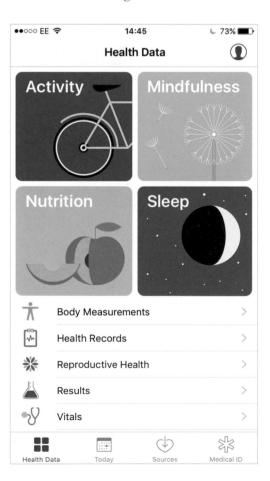

Activity

The Activity category can be used to record various types of activity, from walking to swimming.

1 Tap on the **Activity** button

2 The activity for the current day is displayed below the introductory video. This includes the items that are recorded automatically (**Flights Climbed**, **Steps** and **Walking + Running Distance**). Tap on an item to view its full details and add data as required (see pages 30-32). Swipe down the page to view other activity categories (see the **Don't forget** tip)

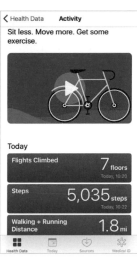

For all of the categories, swipe down the page to see all of the topics within them.

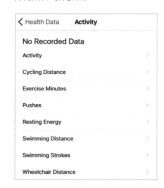

Mindfulness

The Mindfulness category can be used to record times of relaxation and meditation.

1 Tap on the **Mindfulness** button

2 Tap here to watch a short video about mindfulness

3 Tap on the chart to add data about the length of time for your mindfulness activities (this can also be done with bespoke apps from the App Store)

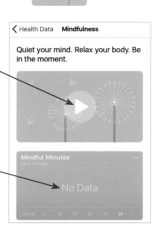
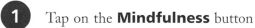

...cont'd

Nutrition

This can be used to record data for a wide range of nutritional topics, from calcium to protein.

1 Tap on the **Nutrition** button

2 Scroll down the page and tap on one of the topics to view its details and add data as required

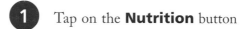

‹ Health Data   **Nutrition**

No Recorded Data

Biotin   ›

Caffeine   ›

Calcium   ›

Carbohydrates   ›

Chloride   ›

Chromium   ›

Copper   ›

Don't forget

Each topic has an appropriate unit of measurement, under the **Unit** heading (once an item has been selected from the list of topics).

Sleep

This can be used to record your sleep patterns:

1 Tap on the **Sleep** button

2 Tap on the **Sleep Analysis** chart to view its details and add data as required. This can be done manually, or with a bespoke sleep app from the App Store

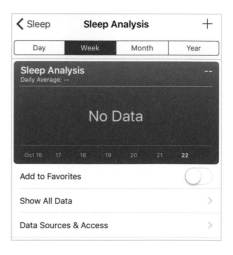

‹ Sleep   **Sleep Analysis**   +

| Day | Week | Month | Year |

Sleep Analysis
Daily Average: --   --

No Data

Oct 16   17   18   19   20   21   **22**

Add to Favorites

Show All Data   ›

Data Sources & Access   ›

Don't forget

The **Sleep** category is best used in conjunction with a sleep analysis app from the App Store, in order to get the most accurate data. Within the Sleep category you can enter the number of hours that you are asleep or awake, but nothing more sophisticated in terms of your sleep pattern.

Body Measurements

This can be used to enter your own Body Measurements.

1 Tap on the **Body Measurements** button

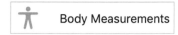

2 Tap on one of the topics to view its details

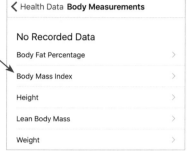

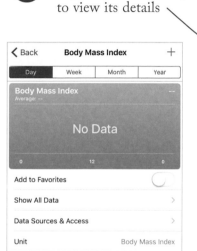

3 As for all categories, tap on a topic to add data for it or view details that have already been added (see pages 30-32)

(see pages 30-32)

Tap on the **Show All Data** option in Step 3 to see all of the details that have been added for the topic, either manually or automatically using the iPhone.

Health Records

This can be used to view and add to your health records from your medical provider (if they provide this service).

1 Tap on the **Health Records** button

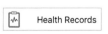

2 If your medical provider has published your health records for your use, tap on the **Show All Records** button to see them, or tap on the **Data Sources & Access** button to select apps with which you want to share your health data

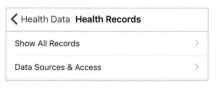

Medical providers have to make your health records available on their website (in Clinical Document Architecture files) in order to access them with the Health app. This is only available with a limited number of medical providers (mainly in the US) but it should expand in time. Ask your medical provider for details.

...cont'd

Reproductive Health

This can be used to record data about pregnancy related topics.

Beware

Do not just rely on the **Reproductive Health** topics if you are concerned about any issues connected with becoming pregnant. Always consult a doctor or a fertility expert in the first instance.

1 Tap on the **Reproductive Health** button

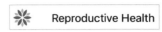

2 Tap on one of the topics to view its details and add data as required

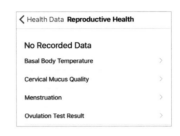

Results

This can be used to record your own health data.

1 Tap on the **Results** button

2 Tap on one of the topics to view its details and add data as required

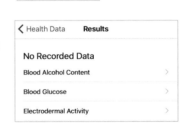

Beware

Always seek professional medical advice if you are concerned about any of the topics in the **Results** or **Vitals** categories.

Vitals

This can be used to record your blood pressure, body temperature, heart rate and respiratory rate.

1 Tap on the **Vitals** button

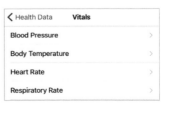

2 Tap on one of the topics to view its details and add data as required

Calendar View

Once health data has been added within the Health app, it can be viewed for the current day or on specific days which are accessed from the calendar. To view health data that has been added for specific days:

1 Tap on the **Today** button on the bottom toolbar

2 The data for the current day is displayed (the current day is indicated by a red circle)

3 Tap here to view the full calendar

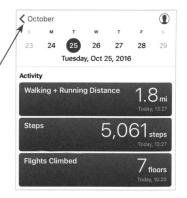

4 Tap on another day on the calendar to view the data that has been entered for that day

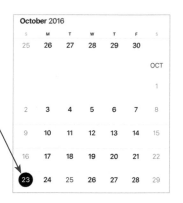

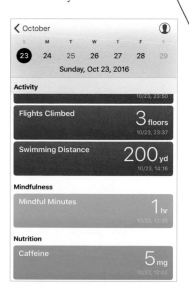

Viewing Health Data

Once you start using the Health app on a regular basis, you will probably find that you use some of the categories and topics more than others, particularly those that calculate your activities automatically through the iPhone, such as Flights Climbed or Steps. To make it easier to view your most popular topics, the Today view within the Health app can be used to display the items you use most frequently. To do this:

Hot tip

The default items on the Today page are those that are recorded automatically by the iPhone and the Health app.

28

Don't forget

If only items from a single category are included in the Today section, all of the panels will be the same color.

1 Tap on the **Today** button

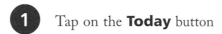

2 By default, the topics for **Walking + Running Distance**, **Steps** and **Flights Climbed** are displayed automatically on the Today page

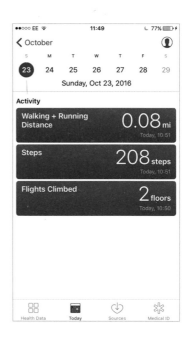

3 If content is added manually for an item, this is then displayed on the **Today** page, underneath the default items

4 Tap on an item on the Today page to view its chart

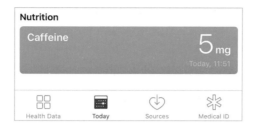

5 Tap on these buttons to view the topic according to the data for **Day**, **Week**, **Month** and **Year**

6 Tap on the chart to view all of the recorded data (or tap on the **Show All Data** button)

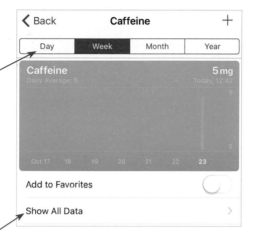

7 Tap on an item to view its full details

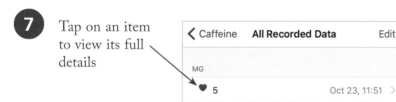

8 The details for each item include the amount recorded, the date of recording and whether it was user entered or not

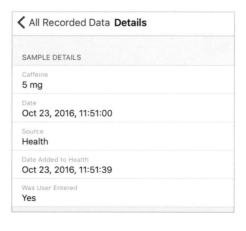

The data for items that are entered automatically and those that are entered manually can be viewed in the same way.

29

Adding Health Data

Except for the items that are added automatically by the iPhone and the Health app (Walking + Running Distance, Step and Flights climbed), each item of health data can be added manually. To do this:

1 Access a topic. At this stage it will display **No Data**

2 Tap on the **+** button to add data for the topic

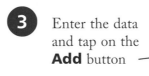

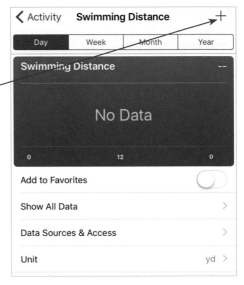

Hot tip

The **Date** and **Time** can also be changed in the window in Step 3.

3 Enter the data and tap on the **Add** button

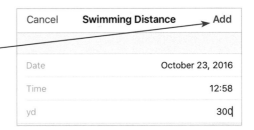

4 The data is added to the chart for the current topic. Tap on the **+** button again to add more data (for the same date)

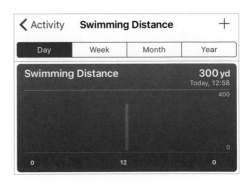

5 Enter more data and tap on the **Add** button again

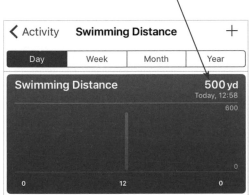

Cancel	**Swimming Distance**	Add
Date		October 23, 2016
Time		12:58
yd		200

6 The chart is updated, including all of the data that has been added for the required date/time period. This way, several items of data can be added for the same day and the aggregated amount is displayed on the chart

< Activity **Swimming Distance** +

| Day | Week | Month | Year |

Swimming Distance 500 yd
Today, 12:58
600
0
0 12 0

7 The items that are added automatically are updated by the iPhone and the Health app, and are displayed on the Today page or under the date on which they were generated

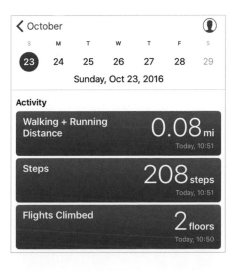

< October

| S | M | T | W | T | F | S |
| 23 | 24 | 25 | 26 | 27 | 28 | 29 |

Sunday, Oct 23, 2016

Activity

Walking + Running Distance — 0.08 mi — Today, 10:51

Steps — 208 steps — Today, 10:51

Flights Climbed — 2 floors — Today, 10:50

Hot tip

It is also possible to add manual data to the items that are automatically updated. Any manual entry is added to the data that has already been generated automatically.

31

...cont'd

Viewing all data

To view all of the items entered for a specific day:

1 Tap on the **Show All Data** option, underneath the chart

Show All Data	>

2 All of the items that have been added are displayed

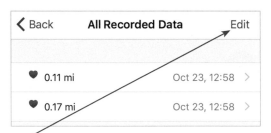

3 Tap on the **Edit** button to select items to delete

4 Tap on this button to delete an item

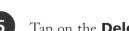

5 Tap on the **Delete** button to remove the item of data

6 The item is removed from the list of data. Tap on the **Done** button to return to the Edit screen

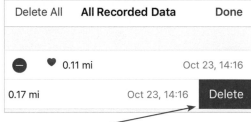

Hot tip

Swipe quickly from right to left on an item of data in Step 2 to access the **Delete** button. Tap on the button to delete the item of data in the same way as in Step 5.

32

Adding Health App Favorites

The Health app items that you use most frequently can be added as favorites so that they always appear at the top of the Today page, or for any date for which they have data entered. To do this:

1 Select a topic and drag the **Add to Favorites** button to **On**

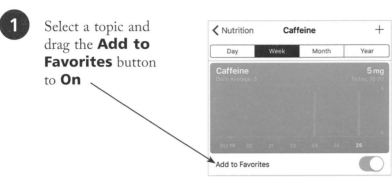

2 Tap on the **Today** button. The item is displayed at the top of the window, beneath the calendar. As more favorites are added, they populate this area in the window

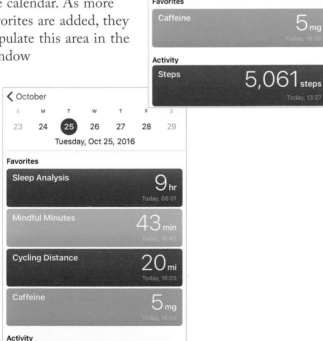

The automatically generated items (Flights Climbed, Walking + Running Distances and Steps) can also be added as favorites.

Sources

The Sources option within the Health app displays apps that have been given permission to access the app and share data with it. To view Sources:

1 Tap on the **Sources** button on the bottom toolbar

Sources

2 Apps that have been given permission to share data with the Health app are listed (permission is usually requested when you first open the app for use)

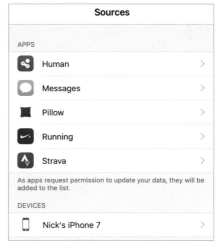

Sources
APPS
Human >
Messages >
Pillow >
Running >
Strava >

As apps request permission to update your data, they will be added to the list.

DEVICES

Nick's iPhone 7 >

Hot tip

Select your iPhone under **Devices** in the Sources section to view details of the items that are collated automatically by the iPhone and stored by the Health app.

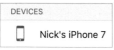

DEVICES

Nick's iPhone 7

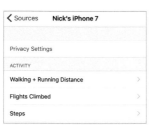

< Sources   Nick's iPhone 7

Privacy Settings

ACTIVITY

Walking + Running Distance >

Flights Climbed >

Steps >

3 Tap on an app to view the range of data that can be shared with it. Drag the buttons **On** or **Off** to share that item of data. Third-party apps can **Write** data, which means that data is sent to the Health app, or **Read** it, which means that it accesses the relevant data from the Health app

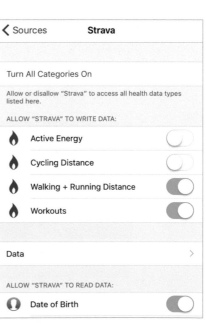

< Sources   **Strava**

Turn All Categories On

Allow or disallow "Strava" to access all health data types listed here.

ALLOW "STRAVA" TO WRITE DATA:

Active Energy

Cycling Distance

Walking + Running Distance

Workouts

Data >

ALLOW "STRAVA" TO READ DATA:

Date of Birth

Medical ID

The Medical ID option within the Health app enables you to enter a range of medical details, which can be used by the app and also by medical professionals, such as in an emergency if they need to obtain certain medical details. To add a Medical ID:

1 Tap on the **Medical ID** button on the bottom toolbar

2 Tap on the **Create Medical ID** button

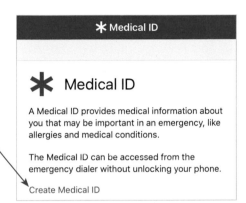

✱ Medical ID

✱ Medical ID

A Medical ID provides medical information about you that may be important in an emergency, like allergies and medical conditions.

The Medical ID can be accessed from the emergency dialer without unlocking your phone.

Create Medical ID

3 Drag the **Show When Locked** button to **On** to display your Medical ID information on the iPhone Lock Screen

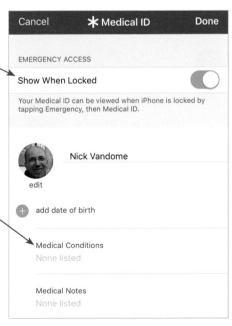

Cancel   **✱ Medical ID**   Done

EMERGENCY ACCESS

Show When Locked

Your Medical ID can be viewed when iPhone is locked by tapping Emergency, then Medical ID.

Nick Vandome

edit

➕ add date of birth

Medical Conditions
None listed

Medical Notes
None listed

4 Tap on items to add medical information to your Medical ID, and then tap on the **Done** button in the top right-hand corner of the window

35

Another option within the Medical ID section is for signing up for organ donation. To do this, tap on the **Add Organ Donor** button and then the **Sign Up with Donate Life** button (or applicable organization for your geographic location, if available).

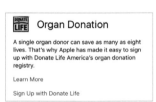

DONATE LIFE Organ Donation

A single organ donor can save as many as eight lives. That's why Apple has made it easy to sign up with Donate Life America's organ donation registry.

Learn More

Sign Up with Donate Life

To view Medical ID information from the Lock Screen, tap on the **Emergency** button (from the Touch ID or Enter Passcode screen) and tap on the **Medical ID** button.

Health App with Apple Watch

The Health app and the Apple Watch can work closely together, so that the data recorded by the Apple Watch can then be viewed, stored and analyzed on the Health app on an iPhone. Once an Apple Watch has been paired and set up with an iPhone (see pages 88-89), it will then share a range of health and fitness information with the Health app on the iPhone automatically. This includes data from the Activity app, the Workout app, the Breathe app and the Heart Rate app. To use the Apple Watch with the Health app:

1 Perform a task with the Apple Watch, such as taking your heart rate with the Heart Rate app

2 Open the Health app on the iPhone

3 Tap on the **Today** button on the bottom toolbar

4 The item from the Apple Watch is displayed under the appropriate heading in the Today section

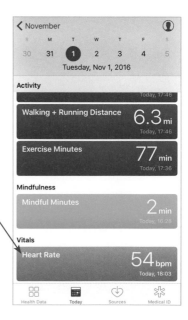

Beware

Your iPhone has to been connected to Wi-Fi or Bluetooth in order for the Apple Watch to share data with it.

5 Tap on the item in Step 4 to view its details. This displays the data chart, which can be viewed according to Day, Week, Month or Year, in the same way as for other items in the Health app

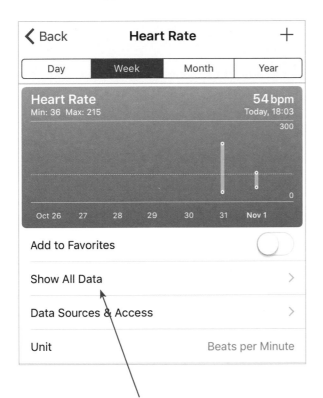

While the data is recorded on the Apple Watch, the best place to view a detailed breakdown of it is on your iPhone.

6 Tap on the **Show All Data** button to view all of the items that have been collated from the Apple Watch. Tap on an item to view a breakdown of the data

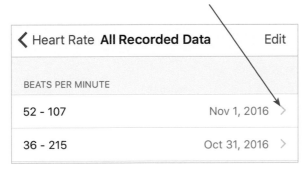

Data from the Activity app on the Apple Watch can also be viewed on the comparable Activity app on the iPhone. See Chapter Seven for more details about using the Activity app.

...cont'd

7 Items with the watch icon next to them indicate that the data has come from the Apple Watch

 54

Beware

If data has been recorded from a different source than the Apple Watch, e.g. another app or the Health app itself, then a different icon will appear next to the data in Step 7.

> **< Back** **All Recorded Data** Edit
>
> BEATS PER MINUTE
>
> 54   Nov 1, 18:03 >
>
> 69   Nov 1, 17:57 >
>
> 73   Nov 1, 17:50 >
>
> 69   Nov 1, 17:47 >

8 Tap on a single item of data to view its details. This includes the date and time at which it was recorded, the source device (e.g. Apple Watch), the time added to the Health app, and details about the device from which it was recorded

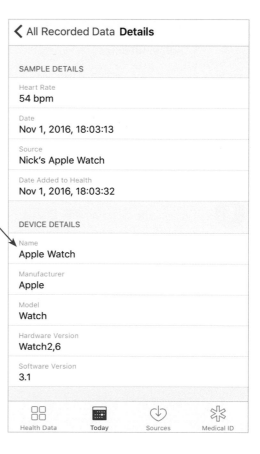

< All Recorded Data **Details**

SAMPLE DETAILS

Heart Rate
54 bpm

Date
Nov 1, 2016, 18:03:13

Source
Nick's Apple Watch

Date Added to Health
Nov 1, 2016, 18:03:32

DEVICE DETAILS

Name
Apple Watch

Manufacturer
Apple

Model
Watch

Hardware Version
Watch2,6

Software Version
3.1

Health Data   Today   Sources   Medical ID

3 Health and Fitness Apps

Apple's App Store has a dedicated category for health and fitness apps. This chapter details how to download these apps, and also covers the range of apps that are available so that you can get started with them, whatever your chosen activity.

Finding Health Apps

Health and fitness is a major global industry, so it is understandable that there is a whole category dedicated to it in the App Store. The Health & Fitness category contains apps that can be used for a range of health and fitness activities: running, fitness workouts, healthy lifestyle and meditation. To find health and fitness apps:

1 Tap on the **App Store** app on your iPhone

2 Tap on the **Categories** button   Categories

3 Tap on the **Health & Fitness** category

App Store	Cancel
⑦ Health & Fitness	✓

4 The **Featured** page of the Health & Fitness category displays the currently featured apps in the top panel, followed by sections for other apps, e.g. Apps for Running

Each category within the App Store has its own Featured page, which is accessed from the **Featured** button on the bottom toolbar.

The items on the Featured page change at regular intervals, as more apps are added.

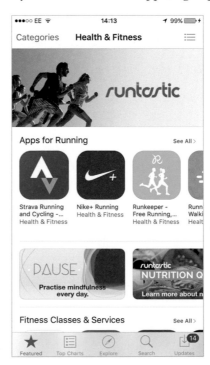

5 Swipe up to see the full range of sections in the Health & Fitness category

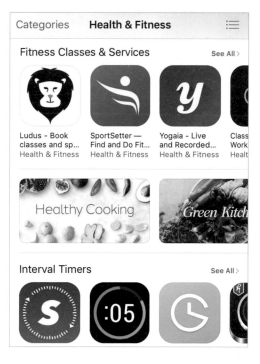

As with web pages, the pages within the App Store move in the opposite direction from the direction of swiping, e.g. if you swipe up, the page moves down, and vice versa.

6 Tap on the **See All** button next to a section to see all of the items within it

7 The apps in each section can be viewed according to **Name**, **Release Date** and **Featured**

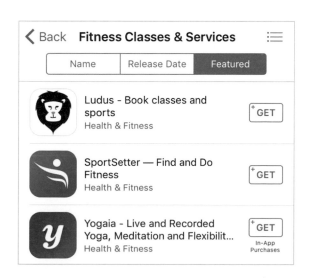

Under the **Name** button in Step 7, apps are displayed in alphabetical order, from A-Z.

...cont'd

Don't forget

The top health and fitness apps can be viewed according to **Paid** apps, **Free** apps and **Top Grossing** apps, which are the ones which have generated the most money in that category in the App Store.

Don't forget

As words are entered into the Search box, suggestions appear below, and these change as you continue typing.

8 To view the top-ranking health and fitness apps, tap on the **Top Charts** button on the bottom toolbar and select the Health & Fitness category as shown in Steps 2 and 3 on page 40

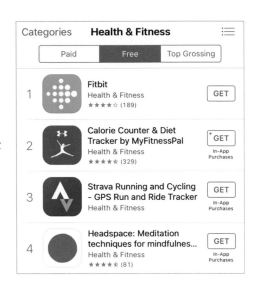

Top Charts

9 To search for specific apps or subjects, tap on the **Search** button on the bottom toolbar

Search

10 Enter the search word or phrase in the Search box. Tap on one of the results

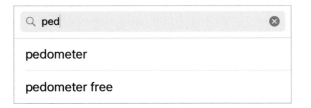

11 View information about the matching apps and download any as required – see the next page for details

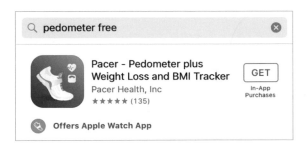

Downloading Health Apps

Once you have located health and fitness apps that you want to try out and use, they can be downloaded from the App Store.

1 Tap on the **Get** (or price) button next to the app's name

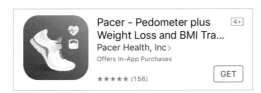

2 Tap on the **Install** button

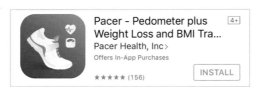

3 Enter your Apple ID password and tap on the **OK** button to start downloading and installing the app

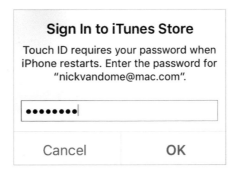

Sign In to iTunes Store

Touch ID requires your password when iPhone restarts. Enter the password for "nickvandome@mac.com".

••••••••

Cancel   OK

4 The progress of the download is displayed next to the app in the App Store

5 The progress of the download is also displayed on the iPhone Home screen

6 Once the download is complete, tap on the app to open it and start using it

Beware

It is worth downloading as many free apps to try as possible. If you do not like an app, just delete it by pressing and holding on its icon on the iPhone Home screen and tapping on the cross in the top left-hand corner.

Don't forget

When downloading apps from the App Store the iTunes Store screen will be displayed when your Apple ID password is required. Touch ID can also be used in this instance, if this is set up.

Don't forget

An Apple ID is required to download apps from the App Store, and to use items from the iTunes Store and iBooks. An Apple ID can be created when you first use one of these apps, or at the Apple website: https://appleid.com

In-App Purchases and Extras

The majority of health and fitness apps are free to download and use. However, a lot of them have extra functionality that has to be paid for. This is known as "in-app purchases". Also, some health and fitness apps require accessories in order for them to utilize their full functionality, e.g. blood pressure measurement apps that require a separate blood pressure monitor.

Locating in-app purchases

If an app provides in-app purchases, this will be indicated next to the app's details in the App Store.

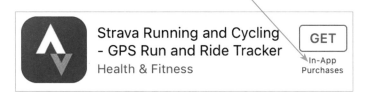

When looking at the details of an app in the App Store, the in-app purchases can be viewed too:

The details of the in-app purchases that are available for an app are usually listed in the app's Details section within the App Store.

① Tap on the **In-App Purchases** button

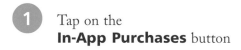

② The in-app purchases that are offered are listed. These cannot be bought through the App Store: as the name suggests, they are purchased through the app itself

Apps can be used perfectly well without in-app purchases, but they usually offer additional functionality, such as comparing your health and fitness achievements with other people.

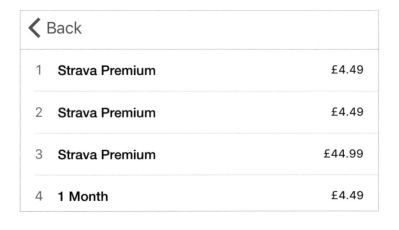

44

...cont'd

From within an app, if there are in-app purchases you will be notified of this when you try to access the paid-for features or from within the app's Settings. For instance, tap on the **Membership** button to view paid-for membership options.

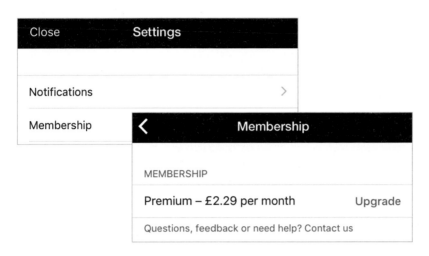

Accessories for apps

For some apps, such as those that measure and analyze body weight or blood pressure, physical accessories are required to record the information in the first place, and this is then displayed within the app. Two of these types of accessories are smartscales for measuring body weight, and wireless blood pressure monitors. These accessories are bought separately, but are usually linked to the company that produces the app for recording the data.

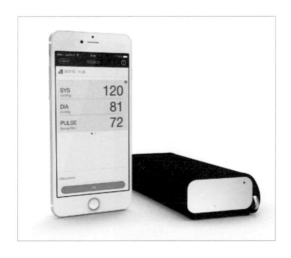

Settings for Health Apps

There are number of different settings that need to be considered when using health and fitness apps. These include the app's own settings, and also those on the iPhone that give it additional functionality, such as Location Services.

Health apps' settings

Each health and fitness app will have its own range of settings:

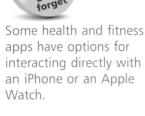

Don't forget

Some health and fitness apps have options for interacting directly with an iPhone or an Apple Watch.

Hot tip

In some health and fitness apps, the **Settings** option is accessed from the **More** button.

1 Tap on this button to access the app's settings

2 The range of settings is specific to each app

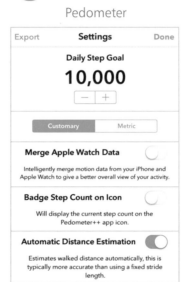

Pedometer

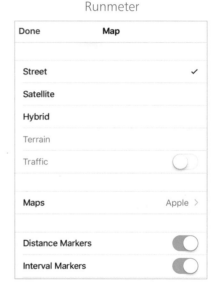

Runmeter

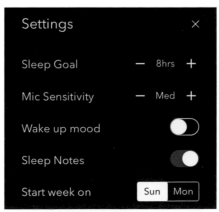

Pillow

iPhone settings

Within the iPhone Settings there are a number of options for how health and fitness apps can access functions on the iPhone that allow them to operate to their full potential. To access these:

1 Tap on the **Settings** app on the Home screen

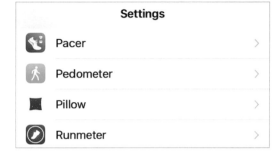

2 Swipe up the list of options in the main Settings panel. Health and fitness apps that have been downloaded will appear here. Tap on one to access its specific settings

The settings for apps that you have downloaded appear below the default settings that are installed on the iPhone.

3 Drag the options **On** or **Off** as required. Tap on the **Location** button to allow or disable Location access

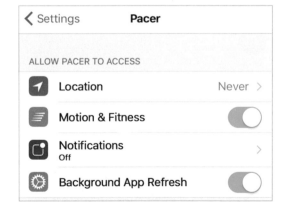

One Location option that is available for some apps is **While Using the App**.

4 Select one of the **Location** options, as required

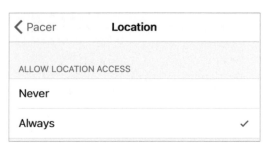

If Location is set to **Never** for an app, it will not be able to use GPS for tracking routes and distances for walking, cycling or running.

...cont'd

Location Services

A number of health and fitness apps use GPS to identify your location so that this can be used for functions such as mapping routes for walking, running or cycling. This can be set up within Location Services in the Settings app:

GPS stands for Global Positioning System and is used to identify someone's location using four or more satellites.

If **Location Services** is turned **Off** in the Privacy section of the Settings app, no apps will be able to use it.

Location Services is used for a range of apps on the iPhone, such as Maps, Calendar and Camera, not just those for health and fitness.

Some apps will prompt you to turn **On** Location Services if it is **Off**.

1 Tap on the **Privacy** button under **Settings**

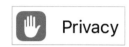

2 Tap on the **Location Services** button

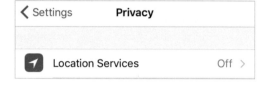

3 Drag the **Location Services** button to **On**

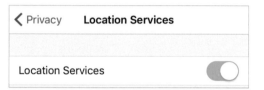

4 Tap on one of the health and fitness apps

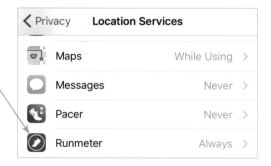

5 Select one of the options for how you want the app to access Location Services on your iPhone

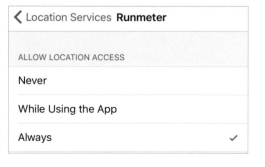

Motion & Fitness sensors

Several health and fitness apps rely on monitoring your movement in order to provide the final data. For instance, for a pedometer app to be able to measure the number of steps that you take each day, it needs to be able to measure your body movement each time you take a step. This is done through the Motion & Fitness sensors, accessed through the Settings app:

Motion in the iPhone is identified by the motion co-processor, in conjunction with the accelerometer sensor.

1 Access **Settings** > **Privacy** and tap on the **Motion & Fitness** button

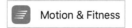

2 Drag the **Fitness Tracking** button to **On**

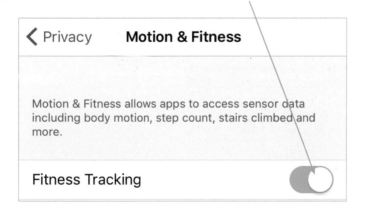

> ‹ Privacy **Motion & Fitness**
>
> Motion & Fitness allows apps to access sensor data including body motion, step count, stairs climbed and more.
>
> Fitness Tracking

Some health and fitness apps will ask for permission to link to the **Motion & Fitness** sensors when they are first opened.

3 Drag the options **On** or **Off** as required for each app

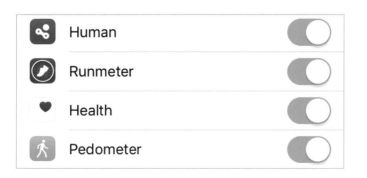

> Human
>
> Runmeter
>
> Health
>
> Pedometer

If Fitness Tracking is turned **Off**, apps that rely on this to monitor motion, such as a pedometer app, will not be able to function.

Pedometer and Running Apps

Walking and running are two of the most common and easiest methods to improve your health and fitness. The App Store contains a range of apps that can be used to record and monitor all of your walking and running needs.

Recording steps and distances

Pedometers and running apps can record your activities in two main ways:

- Recording the number of steps that you take and converting this into distance (step-counter).

- Using GPS on the iPhone to accurately measure distance.

A step-counter app will display the number of steps that you take in a period of time, and show the approximate distance to which this equates. This can be displayed in relation to a daily target. Some step-counter apps also display number of floors climbed, the amount of active time and the number of calories burned.

For a detailed look at walking and running apps, see Chapter Four.

When running with your iPhone, it is a good idea to buy a sports armband for it. This can be used to attach it to your arm, so that you do not have to hold it or have it bumping around in a pocket.

Some walking and running apps can detect when you have stopped and exclude this from your final time, if you are timing your activity.

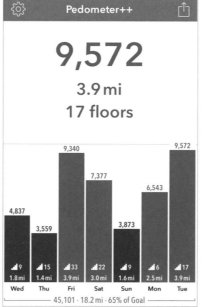

Pedometer

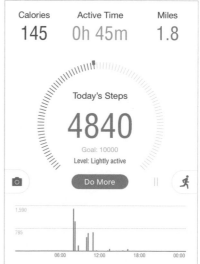

Pacer

An app using GPS will display the distance that you have traveled, measured on a map from your current location. Walking and running data is usually measured in minutes rather than steps.

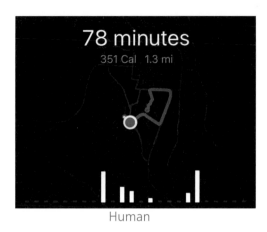
Human

Mapping routes

If you want to work out the distance of a particular route for your walking or running, this can be done by an app for mapping your route. There are several that offer this functionality, using GPS: once you have completed your activity, the route and distance is displayed on a map, so that you know how far you have traveled and the distance, for the next time you do this route. These apps also display the time for the activity. The map of the route can be viewed in its own window.

51

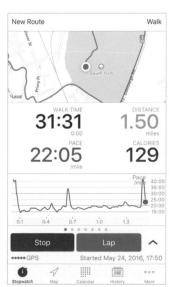

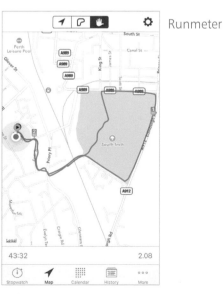
Runmeter

Workout Apps

There are two main types of apps for undertaking workout routines:

- Apps that enable you to book workout classes near to you.

- Apps that can be used to do your own workouts at home.

Apps for finding classes

In the Health & Fitness category of the App Store, there is a Fitness Classes & Services section. The apps here can be used to find fitness and activity classes in your geographical area.

Don't forget

When a fitness classes app is first opened, it will ask to have access to **Location Services** on your iPhone. This has to be accepted in order for the app to use your location and find appropriate classes.

52

1 On the Featured page of the Health & Fitness category, tap on the **See All** button next to the **Fitness Classes & Services** section to see the full range

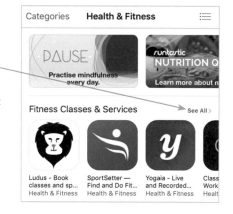

Beware

Only a limited number of organizations are linked to each fitness classes app. If there are no results for classes in your area, this does not mean that there are not any available: try looking online or in the local phonebook instead.

2 Download one of the apps and use it to view and book fitness and activity classes in your own area

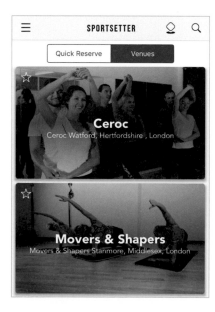

Working out at home

Apps for following workout routines at home are also available in the Health & Fitness section:

1 On the Featured page of the Health & Fitness category, tap on the **See All** button next to the **Quick Routines** section to see the full range

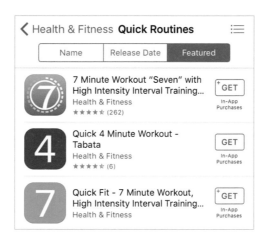

2 Download one of the workout apps and open it from the iPhone Home screen. Workouts can be started by tapping on the **Start** (or equivalent) button. There is also a range of settings that can be specified for the workout (see pages 54-55 for details)

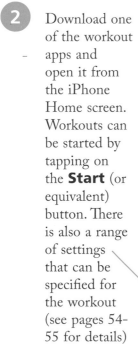

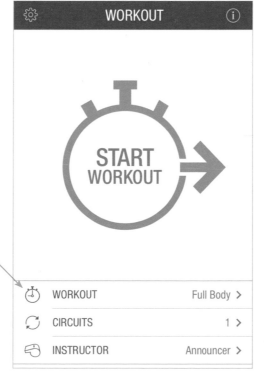

As with a lot of health and fitness apps, workout apps will ask to send you notifications about your progress, and general information about the app. If you do not want to receive these notifications, tap on the **Don't Allow** button.

Prop up your iPhone with a specially designed case, a book, or a similar item, so that you can see it clearly when you are doing your workouts.

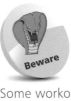

Beware

Some workout apps have in-app purchases for additional types of workouts, in addition to the standard one, which is generally free with the workout app.

 Tap on the **Workouts** button to select the type of workout to be performed

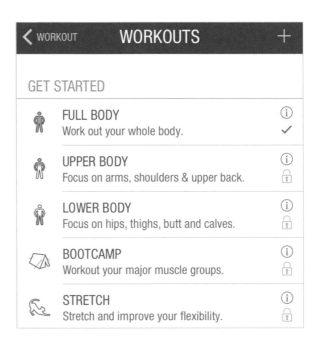

Hot tip

When first starting with a workout app, perform one repetition of the workout and build up from there.

4 Tap on the **Circuits** button to select the number of repetitions for the workout

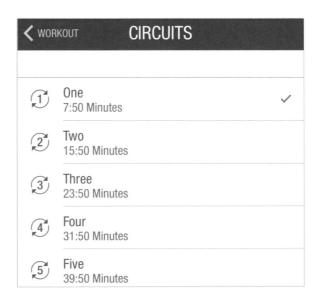

...cont'd

5 Tap on the **Instructor** button to select a gender and voice style for the instructor who accompanies the workout with an audio commentary

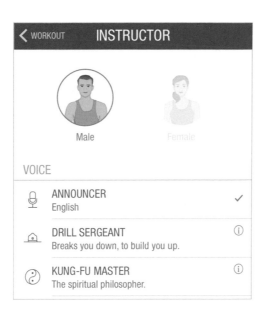

Some instructor voices can be slightly irritating, so experiment with different ones to see which you prefer.

6 Once the workout starts, an animated sequence (or video) displays the exercise to be performed, and the timings for each one. Follow the on-screen action: when one exercise is completed, the app will automatically move on to the next one

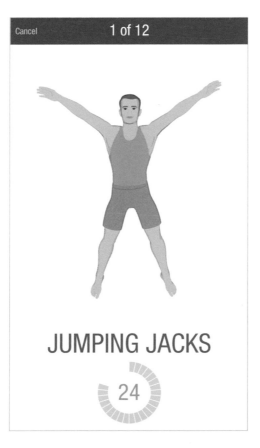

Workout apps also have a rest period of a few seconds between each physical activity.

Yoga and Pilates Apps

Flexibility and agility are important aspects of health and fitness, and can be used together with more aerobic exercises. Yoga and Pilates both offer these, with the added benefit of providing a calming element in terms of relaxation. Yoga and Pilates apps can be searched for within the Health & Fitness category of the App Store, and used to follow a variety of routines:

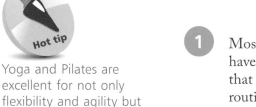

1 Most Yoga and Pilates apps have a selection of videos that can be followed for each routine. Some are provided for free, while additional ones have to be paid for. Tap on a category to view the videos that are available

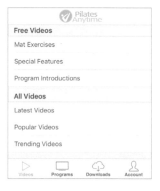

2 Tap on one of the exercises to view the accompanying video

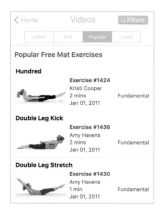

3 Follow the steps in the video to complete the yoga or Pilates exercise routine

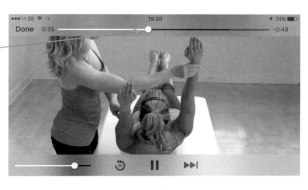

Cycling Apps

Cycling apps are similar to those used to map and measure running activities, except that they are usually used for longer distances. Some apps can be used for both cycling and running. Cycling apps use GPS to map your rides, give distances, and calculate split times and average pace.

1 Before you start your ride you can choose the type of cycling activity that you want to record, e.g. for distance, time, intervals or mountain biking

Cancel	**Select**	Edit

7 Minute Workout
High-intensity circuit training using body weight. Upgrade to Elite for audio cues. See abvio.com/7min for more information.

Cycle ✓

Cycle for Distance
Ride 0.00 miles

Cycle for Time
Ride 0:00

Cycle Intervals
4 times: Ride Fast 1:30, Ride Slow 1:00

Mountain Bike

Rest

2 Tap on the **Start** button to begin recording your cycling route, from your current location. The overall time, distance and speed will be recorded once you have completed your route. Some apps also display the number of calories burned

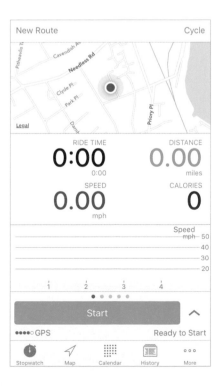

New Route — Cycle

RIDE TIME
0:00
0:00

DISTANCE
0.00
miles

SPEED
0.00
mph

CALORIES
0

Speed mph 50 40 30 20

1   2   3   4

Start

●●●●○ GPS — Ready to Start

Stopwatch | Map | Calendar | History | More

Hot tip

Cycling apps can also automatically break up your route into segments, which are timed individually. You can then try to improve these each time you ride a specific route, and also compare your times with cycling friends on the shared leaderboard.

Don't forget

Cycling apps will ask to have access to your location in **Location Services** in order to map your cycle rides.

Don't forget

Once a route has been mapped and recorded, it is saved within the app, along with the data about the ride. This can then be used as a comparison if you do the same route again.

Golf Apps

Golf is a great way to combine walking and sporting activity, but it is also one of the most technical sports in terms of getting everything in the right place to hit the ball where you want. There are apps that can help you with this, in terms of analyzing your golf swing and comparing it to the professionals:

Beware

Golf can be a frustrating game at times because of its technical nature. However, creating a reliable swing with a golf swing app that you can repeat consistently is an excellent way to ensure that you get as much enjoyment as possible out of playing golf.

Hot tip

Every golfer has their own swing that is unique to them. When comparing your swing with other players, try to take a few pointers from them, without necessarily trying to copy them assiduously.

1 Golf swing apps can be used to video your swing and then analyze it, including the use of color overlays that indicate correct position and direction

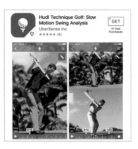

2 Record your swing with your iPhone and play it back with the golf swing app. This can be done in real-time and also in slow motion. This gives you the chance to assess how you can improve your technique and swing. Swing plane drawings can also be placed over your swing for improved analysis

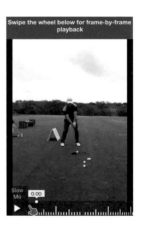

3 Golf swing apps can also be used to compare your own swing to a database of examples from professional golfers

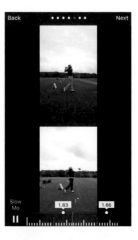

Mind and Body Apps

Developing a healthy lifestyle is more than just physical exercise: a healthy mind can also play an important role in your overall wellbeing. In the App Store there is a range of apps that can help with keeping you calm and relaxed.

1 On the Featured page of the Health & Fitness category, tap on the **See All** button next to the **Meditation & Mindfulness** section to see the full range

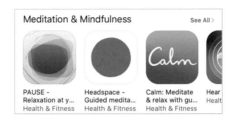

2 Scroll up to view the full range of available Meditation & Mindfulness apps. These cover topics including meditation, improved sleeping and even coloring books for adults

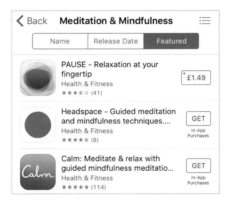

3 Tap on one of the apps to view details about it and tap on the **Get** (or price) button to download the app

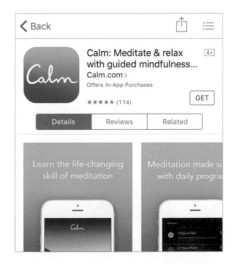

A lot of the Meditation & Mindfulness apps have sections that provide soothing sounds and images, including water scenes, rainfall, bird song and fireplaces.

...cont'd

Meditation apps

Meditation apps offer a number of options for relaxation, in addition to meditation itself. This is what the Calm app offers:

Beware

Some meditation apps have sections for 'Increasing Happiness'. These should be taken with a grain of salt, but improved health and fitness of both mind and body is likely to make you feel more positive about yourself.

Don't forget

Relaxation videos usually come with a soothing background. These can be changed by tapping on the **Scenes** button (or equivalent) within the app.

1 Open the app and select one of the relaxation options and tap on the **Continue** button. (Options can include activities such as meditation, improved sleep and trying to reduce stress and anxiety)

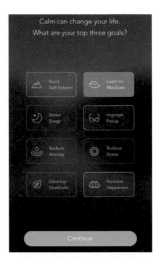

2 Most relaxation options have related videos that contain the relevant content. Tap on the **Play** button to play the content, and follow any instructions

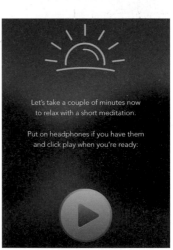

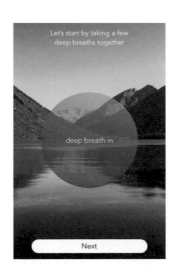

4 Walking and Running

Walking and running are two of the most popular and effective options for keeping fit and healthy. This chapter looks at the types of apps that can be used to record your running and walking routes, including creating new routes, getting feedback as you go, and listening to music.

Calibrating Pedometer Apps

Walking and running are popular and effective ways to get fit and stay healthy. There are several apps for measuring these activities, and they do so in two ways:

● Pedometer apps that count the number of steps you take.

● GPS apps that measure the distance that you travel, including a map of your route.

Pedometer apps use the information from the iPhone sensors (accelerometer, gyroscope and compasses) to enable the co-processors to calculate the number of steps that are taken. This is done through the motion of the iPhone: each step motion is counted as a unit, and the pedometer apps, including the Health App, calculate the number of steps in a given time period, usually a day. The calculation of steps is not 100% accurate, but it gives a fairly good approximation of the number of steps taken.

Working out number of steps

The accuracy of pedometer apps can be tested manually:

● Open a pedometer app and take a note of the current number of steps.

● Walk a specific number of steps, e.g. 100.

● Check the pedometer app to see if there is a disparity between the number of steps taken and the number recorded.

● Repeat the process for a different number of steps, e.g. 200.

● Compare the two figures and calculate any difference.

Once you know any disparity in terms of actual steps and the pedometer figure, you can adjust your targets accordingly. However, the pedometer figure can still be used effectively in terms of comparing daily figures with each other: if the pedometer records 10,000 one day and 11,000 the next day, you know that you have done 10% extra walking or running.

Pedometer apps are not able to calculate stride length, so distance values are only an estimate, albeit reasonably accurate. In order to obtain an exact calculation of distance traveled, a GPS app should be used: it can also be used in conjunction with a pedometer app so that you can compare the distances from the two apps.

When you use a pedometer app, the iPhone needs to be carried with you, either in your hand, in a bag or in your pocket.

If an iPhone is shaken at a steady speed, pedometer apps can sometimes register additional steps.

Pedometer apps tend to slightly overestimate the number of steps taken. However, this could compensate for the times when your iPhone is not counting your steps, e.g. when it is being charged.

Using GPS

GPS stands for Global Positioning System, which uses four satellites with a clear view to locate your geographic location, using your iPhone. With walking and running apps this means that GPS can be used to map the route and distance of your activity with great accuracy. In order for apps to use GPS with an iPhone, Location Services has to be activated for each app. This can be done when you start using the app:

GPS uses a range of satellites in order to pinpoint a location, not just the same four all of the time.

1 When a walking or running app that uses GPS is first opened it will ask for access to your location. Tap on the **OK** button, or

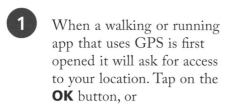

Allow Current Location

Please open the Settings app and allow Runmeter to use your location.

OK

2 Open the **Settings** app and tap on the **Privacy** tab

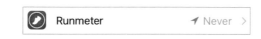 Privacy

3 Tap on the **Location Services** button

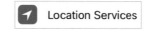 Location Services

If GPS is turned on for the iPhone, this will use more battery power. To turn it off altogether, access **Settings** > **Privacy** > **Location Services** and drag the **Location Services** button **Off**.

4 Tap on the relevant app

 Runmeter   ◥ Never >

5 Select when you want the app to use Location Services, i.e. While Using the App

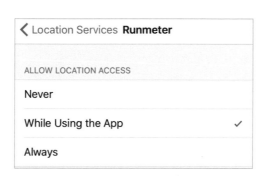

‹ Location Services **Runmeter**

ALLOW LOCATION ACCESS

Never

While Using the App   ✓

Always

6 Once Location Services has been activated for an app this is displayed, as a signal for GPS, within the app

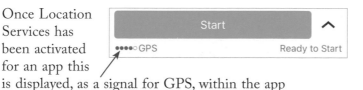

Start   ⌃

●●●●○GPS   Ready to Start

Viewing Distance and Pace

Walking and running apps have differing ways of calculating the distance that you travel and the speed (pace), depending on the type of app; either step-counting pedometer apps or GPS ones.

Pedometer apps

A pedometer app can display an approximation of the distance that you have traveled, based on the number of steps that you have taken. This is not 100% accurate as the app does not know the length of each step. However, it is a useful guide.

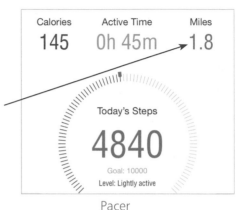

Calories	Active Time	Miles
145	0h 45m	1.8

Today's Steps

4840

Goal: 10000
Level: Lightly active

Pacer

GPS apps

Since GPS apps map and measure the route that you are taking, they can give an accurate display of the distance that you have traveled. This can be done at any stage of the activity, and also at the end with a final reading. GPS apps can also work out the current speed (pace) at which you are moving, and also an average pace once you have finished the activity.

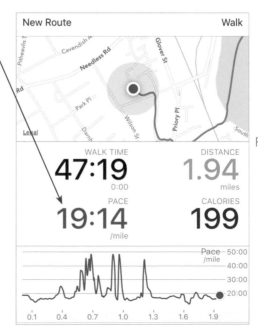

Runmeter

New Route — Walk

WALK TIME	DISTANCE
47:19	1.94
0:00	miles
PACE	CALORIES
19:14	199
/mile	

Key functions offered in walking and running apps are illustarated here using these apps: Human, MapMyWalk, Nike Running, Pacer, Runmeter and Strava.

The unit of measurement for distance traveled can usually be displayed in miles or kilometers, which is selected within the app's Settings.

Some apps can also display your fastest pace.

During a period of activity, you have to be in motion in order for the pace to be displayed.

Burning Calories

Burning calories is one of the reasons why people undertake exercise, and walking and running apps can display the number of calories that have been used, or the amount of energy, for a period of activity. This is an approximation based on the type of activity and any personal information that you have entered into the app, such as gender, weight and height.

1 The number of calories burned, or amount of energy used, is displayed on the readout next to distance and duration

MapMyWalk

> Walked 3.46 km on 5/24/16
> 5/24/16   Walk
>
> Stuart Ave · Needless Rd · Park Pl · Darnhall Dr · Legal · Queen · South Inch · Shore Rd · A989
>
> **DISTANCE**
> **3.46** km
> CALORIES **523**
>
> **DURATION**
> **41:22**
> **STEPS**
> **4694**

Beware

Use the calorie counters in walking and running apps as a rough guide, rather than a definitive figure for the number of calories burned.

2 Tap on the **Energy Burn** button (or equivalent) to select an option

‹ More	Settings	
Distance		Miles ›
Weight		155 lbs ›
Age		51 ›
Gender		Male ›
Energy Burn		Calories ›

Runmeter

3 Tap on one of the options: **Calories** or **Kilojoules**

‹ Settings	Energy Burn	
Calories		✓
Kilojoules		

Runmeter

Don't forget

Some apps ask for your personal details such as weight, height, age and gender, when you first open the app. This information can also usually be entered within the Settings as in Step 2. This information can help the app give a more accurate reading for the number of calories used for a period of exercise.

Viewing Session Data

Every time a walking or running route is completed with a GPS app, the app records and stores the data. This can then be used to view detailed information about that particular session. There is also usually a history option where you can view details of all of the sessions that you have done.

Viewing the most recent session

Once you have completed a session, you can view a range of details about it (this is from the Runmeter app):

The Pace figure in the window in Step 1 shows the pace when you finished the session. This is not an average pace, which is shown in Step 2.

1 The overall details about time, distance, pace and calories are shown on the first screen

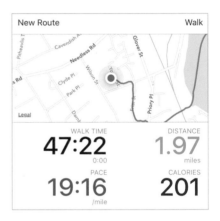

2 Swipe to the left to view the next screen. This shows more detailed information about the pace for the session, including average pace and fastest pace

The ascent and descent figures for a walk or run are calculated by an air pressure sensor in the iPhone 6 or 6s, or later.

3 Swipe to the left to view the next screen. This shows more detailed information about the height that you climbed and descended during the session

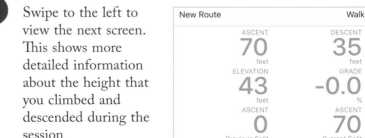

4 Swipe to the left to view the next screen. This shows more detailed information about the number of routes that you have completed

New Route	Walk
YESTERDAY	TODAY
0	**0**
miles	miles
LAST WEEK	THIS WEEK
4	**0**
miles	miles
LAST MONTH	THIS MONTH
4	**1**
miles	miles
LAST YEAR	THIS YEAR
0	**6**
miles	miles

5 Swipe to the left to view the next screen. This shows more detailed information about different segments (splits) of the run or walk

New Route   Walk

Splits

split **1.00 mile**
walk time **29:21**
stopped time **0:00**
average pace **29:21 /mile**
fastest pace **13:39 /mile**
ascent **0**
descent **0**
calories **117**
total walk time **29:21**

split **1.97 miles**
walk time **18:02**
stopped time **0:00**
average pace **18:37 /mile**
fastest pace **12:08 /mile**
ascent **70**
descent **35**
calories **84**
total walk time **47:22**

The segments of a route are generated automatically by the app.

6 Swipe to the left to view the next screen. This shows the overall details of the session

New Route   Walk

ACTIVITY
Walk

WALK TIME
47:22

DISTANCE
1.97 miles

PACE
19:16 /mile

AVERAGE PACE
24:04 /mile

Some of the units of measurement, e.g. miles or kilometers, can be changed within the Settings of most running and walking apps.

...cont'd

Viewing archived sessions

Once a new session of running or walking starts, the previous one is archived in the history section of the app. This means that all of your sessions will be stored so that you can view their data at any time. To do this (in Runmeter):

1 Tap on the **History** button

History

2 Tap on one of the archived sessions to view its details

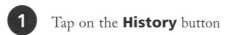

All	
1:00:06	Tue, May 31, 2016
21:22 /mile	New Route
43:32	Tue, May 24, 2016
20:56 /mile	New Route

3 The details of the session are displayed, including the categories on pages 66-67

‹ History	Info ›	Edit

started	May 24, 2016, 17:50
route	*New Route*
activity	Walk
walk time	43:32
stopped time	0:00
distance	2.08 miles
average pace	20:56 /mile
fastest pace	10:30 /mile
ascent	46
descent	41
calories	183

4 Tap on this button to view the collated totals for all of the archived sessions

Σ

Walk		Export

count	2
distance	4.89 miles
walk time	1:43:38
ascent	46
descent	75
calories	436
average distance	2.45 miles
average walk time	51:49
average ascent	23
average descent	37
average calories	218
average pace	21:11 /mile
fastest pace	7:44 /mile

Sharing Details

One way to keep motivated when doing exercise is to share your experiences and achievements with other people. If they do the same, you can create a type of online club where everyone helps to encourage and motivate each other. To share details of your walking and running sessions (in Human and MapMyWalk):

1 To share all of the information for a day's activity, tap on the **Share your day** button

2 The data for the day's activity is displayed (in some apps, you can attach your own photos to this data). Tap on the **Share** button to share the data

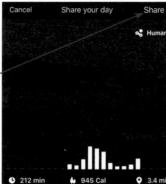

Human

3 Select how you would like to share the details (this can be via email, text or a social media site), or

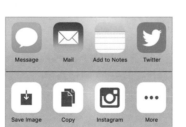

4 For a specific workout session, tap on the **Share** button

MapMyWalk

5 Select how you would like to share the details (this can be via email, text or a social media site)

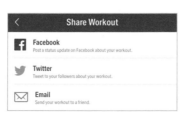

Hot tip

If you have a Facebook account you can link to your friends there and, if they use the same app, compare your times and distances for your activities. For some apps this will require upgrading to a paid-for version of the app.

Hot tip

Joining a local running club is an excellent way to meet like-minded people, take part in group activities and share your experiences and running information.

Creating a Route

When you use a GPS app to map a walk or run, it creates the route that you have taken. By default, this does not have a unique name (except for some apps which use the time and date as the route name). However, it is possible to give a new route a unique name and then select this to follow it again.

To do this (illustrated in Runmeter):

Hot tip

Some apps enable you to stop a session and then restart it by having a Pause and Play/Start button. To finish a session, some apps have a **Done** button.

70

1 Undertake a route by walking or running. This will be displayed on the app's map, with a default name such as New Route. Tap on the **Stop** button to complete the route

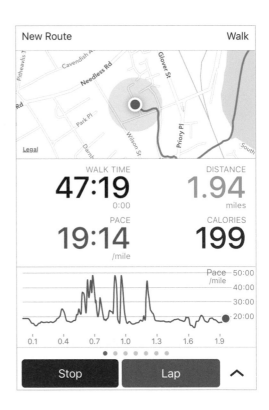

Don't forget

Each time you complete a new route, give it a unique name so that you can easily find it and follow it again.

2 Tap on the **New Route** button   New Route

3 Tap on the **+ / Edit** button

Cancel	**Select Route**	+ / Edit
New Route		✓

4 Tap on the **+** button

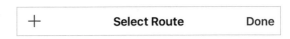

5 Enter a name for the new route and tap on the **Save** button

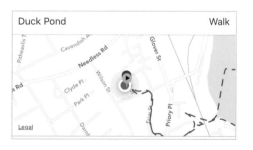

6 The next time you want to walk or run the same route, tap on the **New Route** button and select the route

You do not have to follow the same directions for a completed route if you do it again, but the final data will not be of much use as a comparison.

7 The completed route is indicated by a dotted line

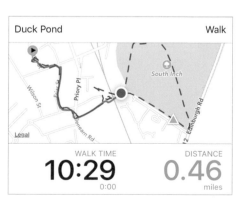

8 Start the walk or run for the route. As you move along the route, the GPS marker can be seen moving along the dotted line (if you are following the same route)

Once you have completed an identical route, you can compare the data in the History section.

Hot tip

If you are using audio feedback during a walking or running session, use headphones on the iPhone so that you do not have to hold it in order to hear the feedback messages.

Don't forget

Audio feedback can inform you about items such as the duration of the workout, distance traveled, average pace, number of steps and calories burned.

Beware

Some walking and running apps require you to upgrade to the paid-for versions in order to get audio feedback.

Using Audio Feedback

Getting a bit of vocal encouragement and information about your workout session is a good way to keep motivated as you are exercising. Walking and running apps have this function in the form of audio feedback, which can be accessed in different ways, according to the app (shown here in Strava):

1 For some apps, the audio feedback is accessed from the **Settings**

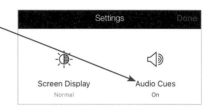

2 Drag the required items **On** or **Off** for audio feedback,

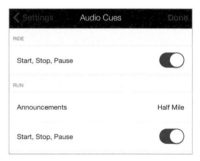

Alternatively, before you undertake a new session (in Pacer):

1 Tap on the **Voice Feedback** button

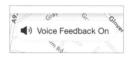

2 Drag the required items **On** or **Off** for audio feedback

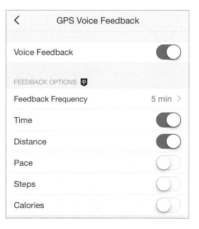

Exercising to Music

One of the best ways to pass the time when doing exercise is listening to music. This can be done by playing music from the Music app, but walking and running apps also enable you to select music that will be played automatically when you start a workout (in Nike Running).

1. For some apps, music can be selected from the **Settings**

2. Select the tracks from the Music app. This can be done by **Playlists**, **Artists**, **Albums** or **Most Played**

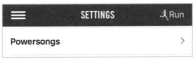

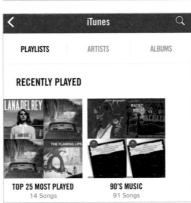

Download music onto your iPhone using the Music app before you play it via a walking or running app. Otherwise, the music will be streamed from the Music app while you are exercising, using your mobile data provider rather than Wi-Fi, which may impact on your data usage limit.

Don't forget

When you start a new workout, any selected music should start playing automatically.

73

Alternatively, before you undertake a new session (MapMyWalk):

1. Tap on the **Music** button

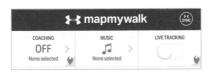

2. Select the tracks from the Music app, in the same way as in Step 2 above

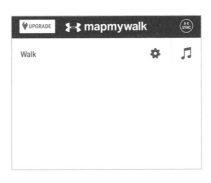

3. Use the music controls within the walking or running app

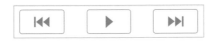

Hot tip

The music controls in the Control Center of the iPhone can also be used to Play, Pause, Rewind, or Fast Forward music that is playing via a walking or running app. Swipe up from the bottom of the iPhone screen to access the Control Center.

Following a Training Plan

Some walking and running apps provide training plans for achieving certain targets such as running a 5K race or a half marathon. If you follow one of these plans, the app will recommend the length of activity for each day. To do this in Runmeter:

Don't forget

Some walking and running apps offer training plans with the free version of the app. For others, it is part of the paid-for version.

Don't forget

If you go over the daily target, the app will still record this and display the data.

1 When undertaking a workout, tap on the type of activity

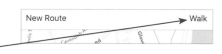

2 Under **Plans**, select the target you want to work towards

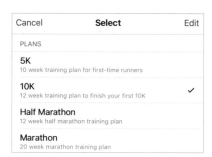

Cancel	**Select**	Edit

PLANS

5K
10 week training plan for first-time runners

10K ✓
12 week training plan to finish your first 10K

Half Marathon
12 week half marathon training plan

Marathon
20 week marathon training plan

3 The plan displays the recommended activity for each day

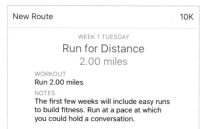

New Route   10K

WEEK 1 TUESDAY
Run for Distance
2.00 miles

WORKOUT
Run 2.00 miles
NOTES
The first few weeks will include easy runs to build fitness. Run at a pace at which you could hold a conversation.

4 Tap on the **Start** button to begin the recommended activity

Start

5 The data for the workout session is specific to the daily target for the activity selected in Step 2

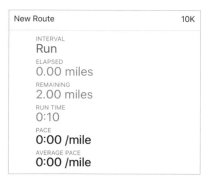

New Route   10K

INTERVAL
Run
ELAPSED
0.00 miles
REMAINING
2.00 miles
RUN TIME
0:10
PACE
0:00 /mile
AVERAGE PACE
0:00 /mile

Coaching plans

Some apps have more in-depth coaching plans that cover a specific period of time leading up to a particular event. These are usually under a Coach heading which gives more tailored advice for each activity (this example is for Nike Running – see pages 85-86 for more details about this app):

1 Tap on the **Coach** button

2 Select a distance for the coaching plan

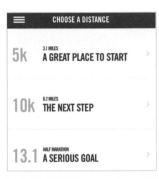

3 Select a level of fitness

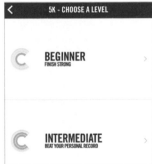

4 Tap on the **Select Program** button

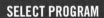

5 Enter details of your race (optional) and tap on the **Start Program** button

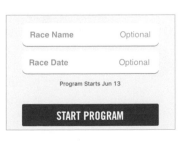

When a coaching program starts, the elements of the whole program will be listed for the recommended time period. This includes days of rest and also non-running or walking activities such as cross-training for stamina.

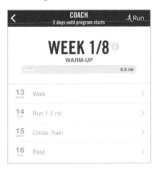

75

More on Featured Apps

There are several walking and running apps in the App Store, all of which perform similar tasks, albeit with some different functions. Also, some apps offer some functions for free, while others only provide the same options in the paid-for version.

Runmeter

This is a versatile GPS app that provides a range of data about each walk or run, and stores it so you can look at the history of your activity.

The items that are in the paid-for version of Runmeter (Elite) include: no advertising; use with Apple Watch; voice feedback; exclude stopped or paused times during a workout; more detailed analysis of your workout data; controlling music during a workout; and sharing your workouts online.

1 Tap on this icon once you have downloaded **Runmeter** from the App Store

2 Tap on the **Stopwatch** button on the bottom toolbar to view the screen for starting a session. Tap on the **Start** button to begin

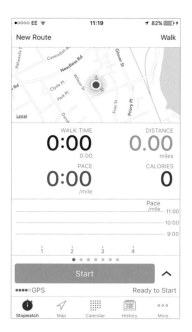

3 Tap on the **Stop** button to finish a session. Swipe to the left in the main window to view information about the session

...cont'd

4 Tap on the **Map** button on the bottom toolbar to view a full-screen map of your latest walk or run

Map

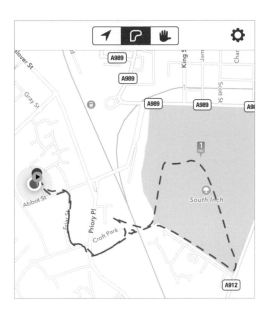

5 Tap on the **Calendar** button on the bottom toolbar to view dates when sessions have been done. Tap on a date to view any sessions for that day, and tap on the session to view its details

Calendar

A green arrow on a date on the calendar indicates the fastest time for a specific route; a red arrow indicates the slowest time. An orange square indicates the median between the fastest and slowest times. A gray dot indicates a time that has been added manually, but for no specific route.

Hot tip

Tap on the **+** button at the top right-hand corner of the calendar to add details of a walk or run manually, for times when you have done a session without your iPhone.

...cont'd

Don't forget

Tap on the totals button on the History toolbar to view the collated data for all of your workouts.

Beware

Items that are grayed-out in the **More** section can only be accessed once the **Elite** version has been purchased.

6 Tap on the **History** button on the bottom toolbar to view all of your archived sessions

History

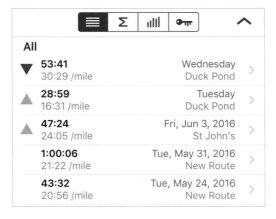

7 Tap on the **More** button on the bottom toolbar to view additional options, including upgrading to the paid-for **Elite** version of the app

More

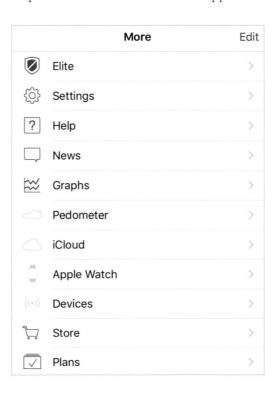

MapMyWalk

MapMyWalk offers similar functionality to Runmeter in terms of tracking and viewing workouts:

1 Tap on this icon once you have downloaded **MapMyWalk** from the App Store

2 Tap on the the **Start Workout** button to start tracking a walk or run

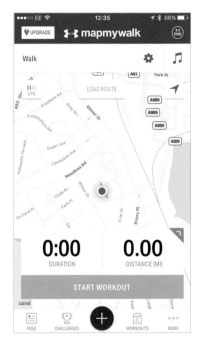

The items that are in the paid-for version of MapMyWalk (MVP) include: no advertising; audio coaching; export workouts; live location tracking; heart rate analysis; custom split times; and training plans.

79

3 Tap on this button to select music to play during the session

4 Tap on this button to select the type of activity for the session

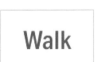

5 Tap on this button to select a specific route, from previous ones that have been undertaken

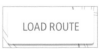

If no route is selected, the session will be recorded with the current date and time.

...cont'd

Don't forget

The options in Step 6 can be accessed from the **+** button on any other screen.

Don't forget

The options in Step 6 include: **Track Workout**, which can be used to start a new workout; **Log Workout**, which can be used to manually enter details of a workout not recorded by the app; **Find Friends**, to link to other friends who are using the app, or invite friends to join via Facebook, Twitter, SMS or email so that you can share workout details; and **Post Status**, to create a post to share about your activities.

6 Tap on the **+** button on the bottom toolbar in Step 2 to access its options

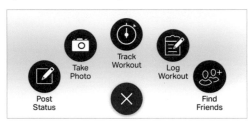

7 Tap on the **Feed** button to access its options, including showing your activities on a timeline that can be viewed by others, and vice versa

8 Tap on the **Challenges** button to set challenges for yourself, or join those set by other people

9 Tap on the **Workouts** button to view workout sessions that you have completed

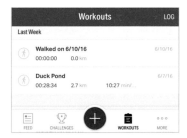

10 Tap on the **More** button to access its options. These include **Settings** and the paid-for **MVP** option

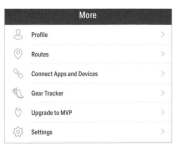

Pacer

This is a step-counter app, which also has a GPS function:

1 Tap on this icon once you have downloaded **Pacer** from the App Store

2 Tap on this button on the bottom toolbar to view the current day's activity for number of steps, calories burned, active time and distance

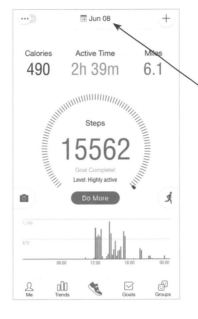

Hot tip

Tap here to access the calendar to view details for different days.

3 Tap on this button in the top right-hand corner of the screen in Step 2 to access the GPS option (see page 82), options for adding your health statistics, and the **Upgrade** option

Don't forget

The paid-for version of Pacer (Upgrade) features: in-depth coaching options; weight loss tracking; and data analysis against global benchmarks.

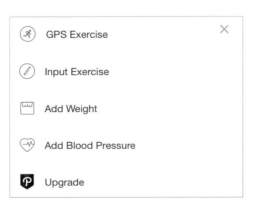

...cont'd

4 Tap on this button from the screen in Step 2 to access the GPS option

5 Select the activity at the top of the screen, and tap on the **Start** button to begin a session that will be tracked by GPS

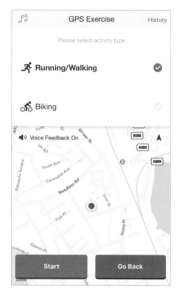

Hot tip

Any GPS walks, runs or cycles recorded in Step 5 can be viewed from the **Me** button on the bottom toolbar.

Don't forget

Tap on the **Goals** button on the bottom toolbar to set your own goals or follow pre-set plans. Tap on the **Groups** button to create your own group for sharing your activities, or join one with like-minded people.

Goals

Groups

6 Tap on the **Trends** button on the bottom toolbar to view daily totals and averages. Swipe to the right to view additional details

Trends

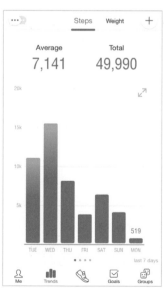

7 Tap on the **Me** button on the bottom toolbar to view your own details in terms of workouts undertaken and archived sessions

Me

Strava

This is a GPS app that is popular with runners and cyclists.

1 Tap on this icon once you have downloaded **Strava** from the App Store

2 Tap on the **Record** button on the bottom toolbar to access the screen for recording a new route, using GPS. Tap on this button to start recording

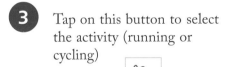

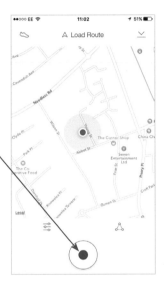

Hot tip

You can create your own routes on the Strava website at **www.strava.com** These can then be accessed from the **Load Route** button at the top of the screen in Step 2.

83

3 Tap on this button to select the activity (running or cycling)

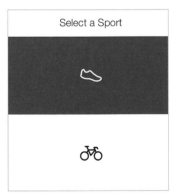

Select a Sport

Don't forget

Tap on this button on the Record screen to access the Settings for this specific area, including **Audio Cues** (audio feedback) and pairing **External Sensors**.

4 Tap on this button to specify settings for any sensors connected to the app

5 Tap on this button to close the Record screen

...cont'd

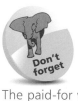

Hot tip

Tap on an item in the Feed section to view any segments that have been created for it. These are sections of a run or cycle that Strava automatically identifies and produces a time for. If the section is done again, another time will be generated, to compare with earlier ones and with other people. You can create your own segments at the Strava website at: www.strava.com

6 Tap on the **Feed** button on the bottom toolbar to view details of your activities. This also includes any friends that you have linked to on Facebook (see Step 8)

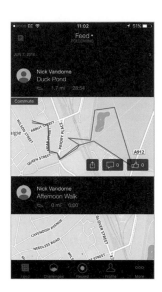

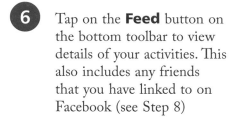

7 Tap on the **Challenges** button on the bottom toolbar to join events that have been added by running and cycling groups

8 Tap on the **Profile** button on the bottom toolbar to access your own details and also link to friends from Facebook

9 Tap on the **More** button on the bottom toolbar to access its options. These include **Settings** and the paid-for **Premium** option

Don't forget

The paid-for version of Strava (Premium) features: personalized coaching; live feedback; and advanced analysis.

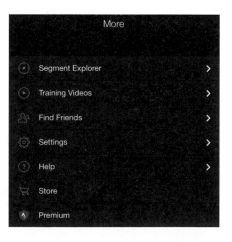

Nike Running

This is Nike's dedicated running app.

1 Tap on this icon once you have downloaded **Nike Running** from the App Store

2 Tap on the **Begin Run** button to start a new run. The data for each run is displayed in real-time in the main window, including details of distance, number of overall runs and average NikeFuel used (see the **Don't forget** tip)

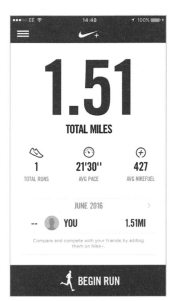

NikeFuel is a Nike invention for measuring all forms of activity. This is done by gaining points whenever you are active. These can be recorded using various Nike apps, with the best overall one for NikeFuel being Nike Move. Overall NikeFuel scores can also be shared and compared with other people.

3 Tap on this button to access the app's menu. Tap on the **Home** button at any point to go back to the screen in Step 2

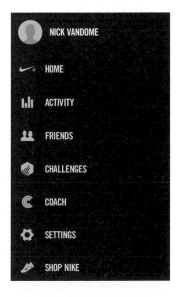

Tap on the **Coach** button on the main menu to access tailored coaching plans for specific distances (see page 75).

85

...cont'd

Hot tip

Tap on these icons on the activity page to, from left to right, rate your run and specify the surface on which it was carried out.

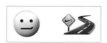

Don't forget

Tap on the **Challenges** button on the main menu and tap on the **Start a New Challenge** button to create a new challenge and invite friends to do it with you.

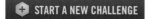

4 Tap on the **Activity** button on the main menu to view your running activity. Tap on the **+** button to add details of a new run manually

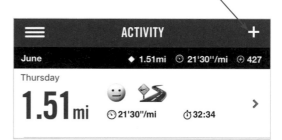

5 Tap on a session in Step 4 to view it on a map

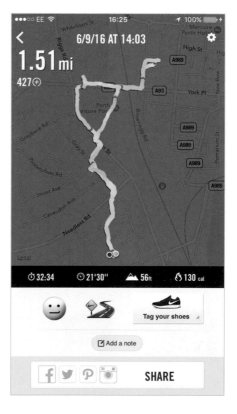

6 Tap on the **Friends** button on the main menu to share run details with selected friends, using the **Find & Invite Friends** button

FIND & INVITE FRIENDS

5 iPhone and Apple Watch

The Apple Watch is designed to be an important companion to you when you are undertaking exercise. This chapter shows how to set it up, and covers its settings and the built-in apps that come with it.

Pairing the Apple Watch

The Apple Watch works best as a companion to the iPhone (5s or later) so that information can be shared between the iPhone and the Apple Watch. Therefore, the first thing to do with the Apple Watch is to 'pair' it with the iPhone so that they can communicate with each other. To do this:

1 Turn on the Apple Watch (see page 90) and tap on the **Watch** app on the iPhone

2 Tap on the **Start Pairing** button

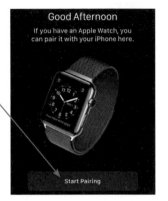

Hot tip

The Apple Watch can also connect to the iPhone using a cellular 3G/4G connection.

3 Turn on Wi-Fi and Bluetooth on the iPhone (**Settings** > **Wi-Fi/ Bluetooth**) and tap on the **OK** button

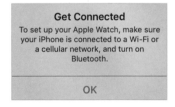

Hot tip

There is also a Bluetooth option in the Settings app on the Apple Watch. However, this is for pairing other devices, such as Bluetooth headsets, and does not affect pairing with the iPhone.

4 When the pairing is completed, tap on the **Set Up Apple Watch** button to continue setting up the Apple Watch (see next page)

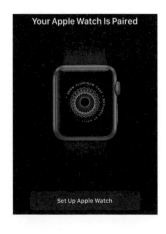

Setting Up the Apple Watch

After the Apple Watch has been paired with an iPhone, some other settings can be applied before it is ready for use.

- **Wrist selection**. Tap on the **Left** or **Right** button to select the wrist on which you want to wear the Apple Watch.

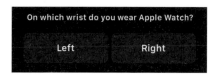

- **Workout Route Tracking**. This can be used to let the Apple Watch use your location to track a workout route and provide local weather information. Tap on either **Enable Route Tracking** or **Disable Route Tracking**.

- **Diagnostics**. This can be used to automatically send Apple details about your Apple Watch use and any issues, to improve its performance. Tap on either **Automatically Send** or **Don't Send**.

- **Shared Settings**. This can be used to share settings for Location Services, Find My iPhone, Siri, Wi-Fi calling, and diagnostics. Tap on the **OK** button.

- **Apple Watch Passcode**. This can be used to create a passcode that can be used to unlock the Apple Watch if it is taken off. The passcode is required to use it again, therefore making it more secure if you lose it or if it is stolen.

- **Activity**. This can be used to enter information about yourself that can be used by the Activity app. This includes your birthdate, gender, height, weight, and if you are a wheelchair user or not. Tap on the **Set up Activity** button, add the information (see Chapter Seven) and tap on the **Continue** button. It is also possible to enter your goals for the categories within the Activity app.

- **Install Available Apps**. Some apps on the iPhone also have versions that are compatible with the Apple Watch. This option can be used to install all compatible apps automatically. Tap on either **Install All** or **Choose Later**.

When the settings have been applied, the Apple Watch will sync with the iPhone and be ready for use.

The Activity goals are those that appear as the daily goals within the app. Enter these as required, or accept the defaults.

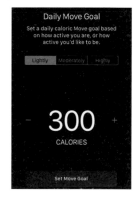

Some of the setup options can be skipped and enabled at a later time, through the **Settings** app on the Apple Watch or the **Watch** app on the iPhone, see pages 98-105 for details.

Around the Apple Watch

The Apple Watch is a stylish smartwatch that can be used to interact with an iPhone and collate a range of health and fitness information to help you achieve your goals in these areas. The elements of the Apple Watch include:

The Digital Crown can be used to navigate around the Apple Watch and select items.

Press and hold the Side button to turn the Apple Watch **On**.

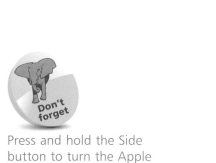

There are two sensors each for the heart and accelerometer functions (opposite each other). The accelerometer sensors can be used to measure your movements, and the data is then used by the Activity and Workout apps for their various functions.

Digital Crown   Side button

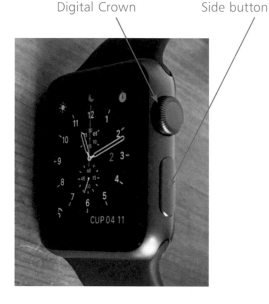

Strap release button   Speaker

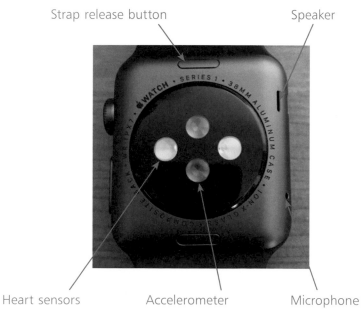

Heart sensors   Accelerometer   Microphone

To use the Apple Watch:
Some of the functionality of the Apple Watch includes:

1 From the Home screen, tap on
an item on the screen to open it
(press the Digital Crown to go
back up a level)

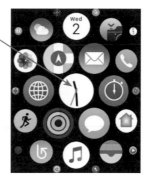

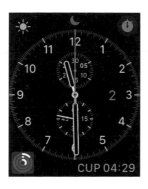

Tap on any app on the
Home screen to make it
the active one. Tap on
this app to access the
current Watch Face.

2 If there is more information
than can be displayed on the
screen, turn the Digital Crown
to view the rest of the screen
(the progress bar shows a green
bar), or

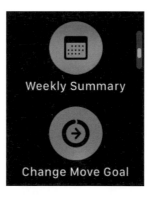

Weekly Summary

Change Move Goal

Press firmly on the
Watch Face to access
other faces and options
for customizing the
current one. See pages
114-115 for more details
about using Watch Faces
on the Apple Watch.

3 Swipe up and down with your
finger on the face of the Apple
Watch to move up and down a
screen (the progress bar shows
a white bar instead of a green
one)

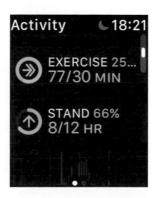

Activity   ☾18:21

EXERCISE 25...
77/30 MIN

STAND 66%
8/12 HR

When the Apple Watch
is on, press the Side
button once to access
the Dock, see page 93.

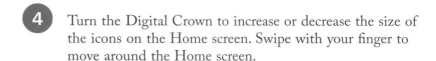

...cont'd

Position an app's icon in the middle of the Home screen and keep turning the Digital Crown to open the app.

92

The Control Center and the Notification Center can only be accessed from a Watch Face screen. They cannot be accessed from other apps or the Home screen.

4 Turn the Digital Crown to increase or decrease the size of the icons on the Home screen. Swipe with your finger to move around the Home screen.

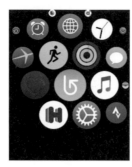 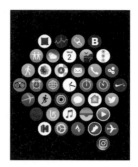

5 Swipe up from the bottom of any Watch Face screen to view the Control Center. This displays Battery charge, Airplane Mode, Silent Mode, Do Not Disturb, Pinging iPhone (to ensure it is connected), and AirPlay

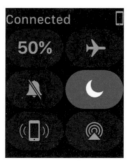

6 Swipe down from the top of any Watch Face screen to access the Notification Center

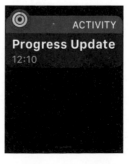

7 Press the Side button once to view the Dock. This contains thumbnails of commonly used apps

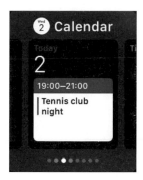

Hot tip

There is a Settings app for the Apple Watch and settings can also be applied from the Watch app on an iPhone. Settings can be applied here for a range of items, including what appears in Notifications and the Dock. See pages 94-97 for more information about using Settings.

8 Swipe left or right to view the apps on the Dock. Tap on one to make it the currently active app. (Press once on the Side button to exit the Dock)

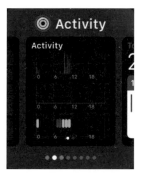

9 Press and hold the Side button and tap on the **Power Off** button to turn off the Apple Watch

Hot tip

Press and hold the Digital Crown to activate Siri, the digital voice assistant. See pages 116-117 for more details.

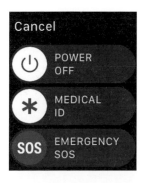

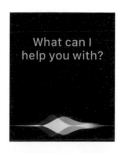

Settings on the Apple Watch

The settings for the Apple Watch can be applied from the Apple Watch itself and also from the Watch app on the iPhone (there are a greater number of options within the Watch app settings). To use the Apple Watch Settings:

Don't forget

Tap on a setting to view its options.

1   Tap on the **Settings** icon on the Home screen

2   Swipe down the screen, or use the Digital Crown to scroll, to view all of the settings on the Apple Watch

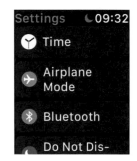

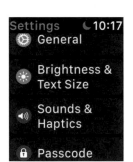

Don't forget

If Airplane Mode is turned **On**, the Apple Watch will not be able to use any network communications, i.e. Bluetooth, to communicate with your iPhone. On a plane, your iPhone should also have Airplane Mode activated.

3   Tap on the **Time** setting to manually change the display on the Watch Face (this does not change the time of any notifications or alerts)

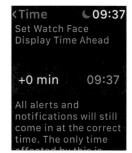

4   Tap on the **Airplane** setting to turn Airplane Mode **On** or **Off**

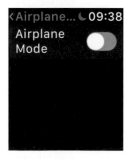

94

5 Tap on the **Bluetooth** setting for the Apple Watch to search for Bluetooth devices in range. (This is used to connect to other Bluetooth devices, such as Bluetooth headphones, not the iPhone. When Bluetooth is turned On on the iPhone, this connects both devices)

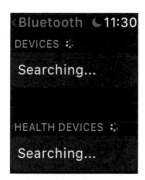

6 Tap on the **Do Not Disturb** setting to turn this **On** or **Off**

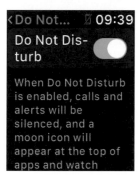

At the bottom of the list of General settings are ones for **Regulatory**, which provides regulatory information about the Apple Watch for different regions, and **Reset**, which returns the Apple Watch to its factory settings and removes any content and settings, including Activation Lock, if it has been set.

7 Tap on the **General** setting to access the options here. They include: **About**, for general information about the Apple Watch; **Orientation**, for the wrist on which the watch is worn and the way in which the Digital Crown faces; **Wake Screen**, for waking the Apple Watch when the wrist is raised; **Wrist Detection**, for locking your Apple Watch when you are not wearing it (if a passcode is used); **Nightstand Mode**, to display the time horizontally if the Apple Watch is being charged on its side; **Accessibility**, for vision accessibility settings; and **Siri**, for enabling Hey Siri, so that the digital voice assistant can be used by saying this

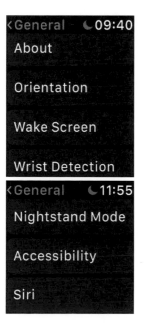

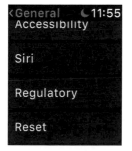

...cont'd

8 Tap on the **Brightness & Text Size** setting to access options for changing the screen brightness and the text size. Drag this slider to alter the screen brightness of your Apple Watch

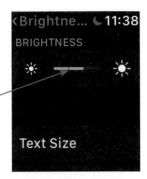

9 Tap on the **Text Size** button to change the size of text in apps that support Dynamic Type, which allows for text to be enlarged or reduced as required

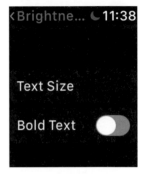

10 Drag the **Bold Text** setting button **On** or **Off** to enable or disable this on your Apple Watch

11 Tap on the **Sounds & Haptics** setting to access options for changing the volume for alerts on the Apple Watch, or putting it into Silent Mode

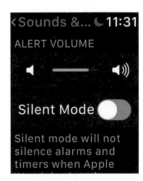

12 Swipe or scroll down the Sounds & Haptics screen to view options for using the Haptic options on the Apple Watch. Tap here to change the strength required to activate a Haptic option. Drag the **Prominent Haptic** button to **On** to create a vibration and play a sound for certain notifications

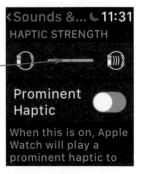

13 Swipe or scroll down the Sounds & Haptics screen and tap the **Tap to Speak Time** button **On** or **Off** to enable the Mickey and Minnie Mouse watch faces to speak the time when you tap on them

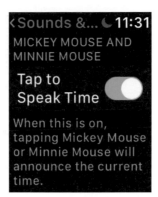

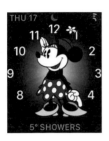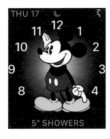

For more details about changing and customizing Watch Faces, see pages 114-115.

14 Tap on the **Passcode** setting to set a passcode that must be entered to unlock the Apple Watch if it has been taken off your wrist

A passcode has to be used if you want to use Apple Pay on your Apple Watch.

15 Swipe or scroll down the Passcode screen to view whether **Unlock with iPhone** is **On** or **Off**. This has to be set up on the iPhone, and if it is **On**, the Apple Watch will be unlocked when the iPhone is unlocked (if you are wearing the Apple Watch and it has a passcode)

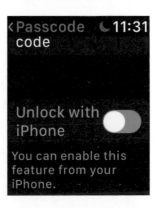

Settings on the Watch App

Settings for the Apple Watch can also be applied from the Watch app on your iPhone. There is a greater range of settings here, and also options for managing Watch Faces. To use Apple Watch settings from the Watch app:

1 Tap on the **Watch** app on your iPhone

2 Tap on the **My Watch** button on the bottom toolbar

3 Tap on the options and settings within the My Watch section. These include information about the Apple Watch, managing Watch Faces, system settings for the Apple Watch and also those for specific apps

Other sections within the Watch app are **Face Gallery**, for adding more Watch Faces, **App Store**, for downloading more Apple Watch compatible apps, and **Search**, for searching for Apple Watch compatible apps in the App Store.

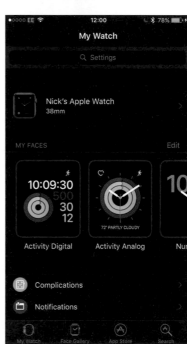

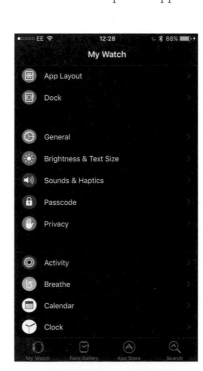

...cont'd

Apple Watch details

To view information about your Apple Watch:

1 Tap on the name of your Apple Watch at the top of the **My Watch** section

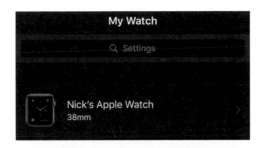

The name of your Apple Watch is the one that you gave to it when it was first set up.

2 Details about the Apple Watch are displayed, including an option to **Pair a new Apple Watch**. Tap on this button to view further options

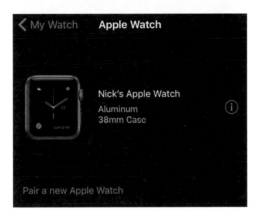

3 Tap on the **Find My Apple Watch** button to locate a lost Apple Watch. Tap on the **Unpair Apple Watch** to unpair it from your iPhone

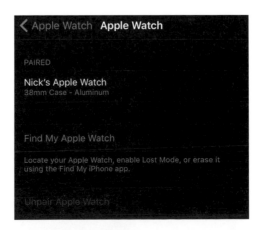

The **Find My Apple Watch** function uses the Find iPhone app on your iPhone to display the location of your Apple Watch on a map, when you tap on the button in Step 3.

...cont'd

Editing Watch Faces
To edit the current Watch Faces on the Apple Watch:

1 Tap on the **Edit** button on the **My Faces** panel in the **My Watch** section

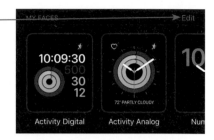

Hot tip

New Watch Faces are developed on a regular basis and are often issued when there is an update to the Apple Watch operating system, WatchOS. If there is an update for this, it can be installed from the Watch app on your iPhone.

2 The Watch Faces that are currently available for the Apple Watch are displayed. Tap on the red circle and tap **Remove** to delete one

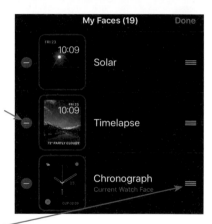

3 Press on this button next to a Watch Face and drag it into a different position to change the order in which they appear on the Apple Watch when switching Watch Faces

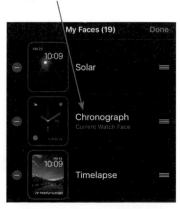

System settings

The system settings for the Apple Watch from within the Watch app include:

Complications. This can be used to add different elements (complications) to Watch Faces. The third-party apps that support this are listed in the Complications section.

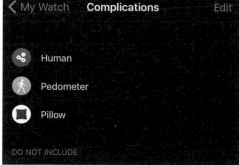

Complications can be added to the Utility or Modular Watch Faces. To do this, press on the relevant Watch Face until it vibrates, and then tap on the **Customize** button. Swipe to the left to the final screen and tap on one of the elements (complications). Use the Digital Crown to scroll through options for the selected element. Press the Digital Crown to return to the Customize screen and press it again to return to the original Watch Face.

Notifications. This can be used to determine how notifications are handled by the Apple Watch:

1 Drag the **Notifications Indicator** button to **On** to display a red dot at the top of the Watch Face when there is a new notification

2 Tap on individual apps to specify how they deal with alerts

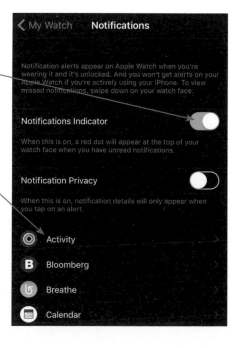

One of the options for individual apps is to **Mirror my iPhone** (for compatible apps). If this is checked **On** (indicated by a tick next to it), the notification settings will be applied to the Apple Watch too.

...cont'd

App Layout. This can be used to edit the layout of how apps appear on the Apple Watch:

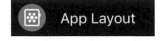

1 The current layout is displayed when you tap on the **App Layout** button

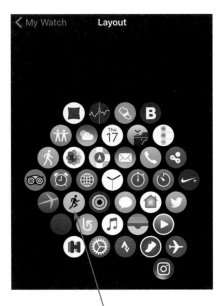

Hot tip

Most system apps cannot be removed from the Apple Watch, but some third-party ones can be removed. See page 109 for details.

2 Press and hold on an icon and drag it into a new position in the layout. This will be replicated on the Apple Watch

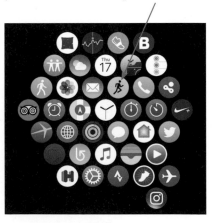

...cont'd

Dock. This can be used to determine the items that appear when the Dock is accessed on the Apple Watch:

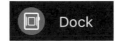

① The current layout is displayed when you tap on the **Dock** button

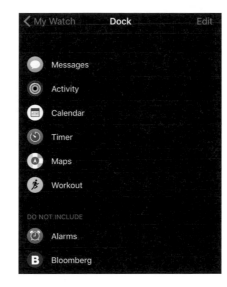

② The items currently available from the Dock are listed at the top of the panel. Those that can be added are listed under **Do Not Include**

Don't forget

The Dock is accessed on the Apple Watch by pressing the Side button once.

③ Tap on the **Edit** button at the top of the window to edit the Dock items

④ Tap on the red circle next to one of the Dock items and tap on the **Remove** button to remove it from the Dock. Tap on the green circle next to one of items under **Do Not Include**, to add it to the Dock

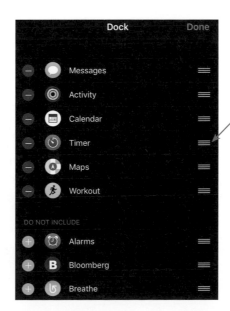

Hot tip

Press and hold on this button next to a Dock item to drag it into a different position on the list. This will also change the order on the Dock itself on the Apple Watch.

General. This includes an expanded range of settings to those found on the Apple Watch:

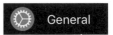

Apps must have a compatible Apple Watch version for them to be installed as in Step 1.

1 Drag the **Automatic App Install** button to **On** to automatically sync your iPhone apps with your Apple Watch

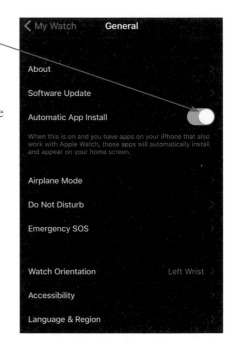

2 Tap on the other General options to apply settings as required

Brightness & Text Size. This has similar options as for the same setting on the Apple Watch, for changing the screen brightness, the text size and using bold text in compatible apps.

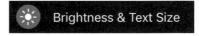

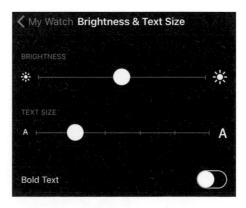

Sounds & Haptics. This has similar options as for the same setting on the Apple Watch:

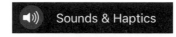

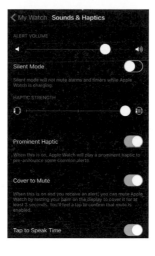

1 Drag the **Cover to Mute** button to **On** to Mute the Apple Watch when you receive an alert, by placing your hand over the Apple Watch for at least three seconds

The **Alert Volume** option is the same as the one in the Sounds & Haptics settings on the Apple Watch. However, the scale on the Watch app is larger, giving more accuracy when setting the alert volume.

Passcode. This has options for creating a passcode, turning off a passcode, changing a passcode, using a 4-digit passcode, unlocking your Apple Watch when you unlock your iPhone, and erasing the data from your Apple Watch.

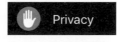

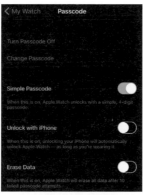

Privacy. This has an option for sharing the Motion & Fitness settings from your iPhone to your Apple Watch. This includes using your heart rate to calculate calories burned, and your body movement to determine your step count and fitness level.

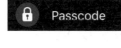

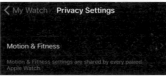

Built-in Apps

There are several apps that come built-in with the Apple Watch. Some of them mirror the same app on your iPhone, and their settings can be applied within the Watch app on the iPhone.

Apps can be downloaded to your Apple Watch from the Watch app on your iPhone, see pages 145-146 for details.

To ensure an app on your Apple Watch mirrors the same one on your iPhone (if it has this functionality), access the **Watch** app on the iPhone and tap on the **My Watch** button on the bottom toolbar. Swipe down the page, tap on the required app, and tap **On** the **Mirror my iPhone** option so that an orange tick appears next to it.

- **Activity**. This app measures your activity, using three criteria: Move, Exercise and Stand. See Chapter Seven for details.

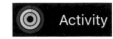

- **Breathe**. This app can be used to remind you to pause during the day and do some relaxing breathing.

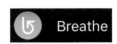

- **Calendar**. This app can be used to mirror the Calendar app on your iPhone and display the same information. If an item is added on your iPhone, it will show up on this app on your Apple Watch.

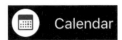

- **Clock**. This covers the Watch Faces that are used to view the time. There are also apps for a World Clock, a Timer and a Stopwatch.

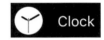

- **Contacts**. This app can be used to mirror the Contacts app on your iPhone and display the same information. If an item is added on your iPhone, it will show up on this app on your Apple Watch.

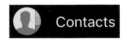

- **Health**. Although this is not a specific app on the Apple Watch, there are settings for it that can be applied through the Watch app on the iPhone.

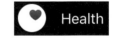

- **Mail**. This app can be used to mirror the Mail app on your iPhone and display some of the same information. It can be used to view emails and send replies, although the functionality is more limited than with the Mail app on the iPhone.

- **Maps**. This app can be used to view your location and get directions to different locations. See pages 122-124 for details.

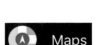

● **Messages**. This app can be used to mirror the Messages app on your iPhone and display the same information. It can be used to view and reply to messages. See pages 118-120 for details.

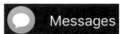

● **Music**. This app can be used to select and play music, either through the Apple Watch or on the iPhone.

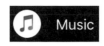

● **Phone**. This app can be used to receive calls and respond to them. It can display an incoming call and allow you to reply to it via your Apple Watch, send an automated response, or take the call on your iPhone.

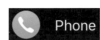

If you answer a phonecall with your Apple Watch, everyone around you will be able to hear both sides of the conversation, unless you are using a Bluetooth headset for the call.

● **Photos**. This app can be used to view photos that have been taken with the Apple Watch Camera app, or specific albums that have been synced from the Photos app on the iPhone. See pages 125-126 for details.

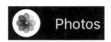

● **Stocks**. This app can be used to display prices for up to 20 stock prices. These stocks can be added to the Stocks app on the iPhone, which will then appear in the app on the Apple Watch.

● **Wallet & Apple Pay**. This app can be used to add debit and credit cards to the Apple Watch so that it can use the contactless payment system, Apple Pay. See pages 128-129 for details.

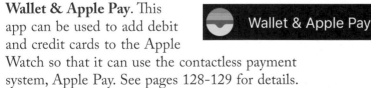

The built-in apps listed here are the ones which have related settings in the Watch app on the iPhone. Other built-in Apple Watch apps are Reminders, Camera, Home (for controlling compatible items in the home, such as heating controls) and the Settings app.

● **Weather**. This app can be used to display weather forecasts for locations around the world. Locations cannot be added from the Apple Watch, but the app mirrors the locations added to the companion Weather app on the iPhone.

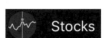

● **Workout**. This app can be used to record specific periods of workout activity. See Chapter Eight for more details.

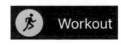

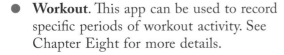

Individual App Settings

Within the My Watch section of the Watch app, settings can also be applied for individual apps, as well as the system settings.

Don't forget

Some of the apps on the Apple Watch are built-in ones and some are added from the App Store. For built-in apps, one of the commonly used settings is **Mirror my iPhone**. This can be used to sync the information on your iPhone and Apple Watch, for compatible apps.

1 Scroll down the screen in the **My Watch** section to view the individual apps

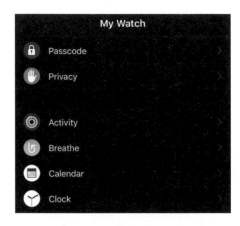

2 Tap on an app to view its available settings

3 The settings differ for each app. Drag the buttons **On** or **Off** to apply a setting or tap on an item to view more details about it

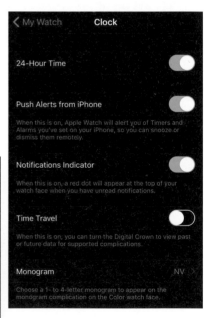

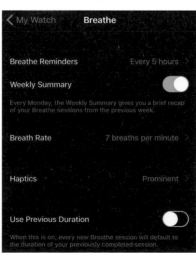

Hiding Apps

Some of the apps on the Apple Watch are built-in ones that cannot be removed. However, some other apps can be hidden from view; generally ones that have been downloaded from the App Store. To hide an app with the Watch app on your iPhone:

1 Scroll down the screen in the **My Watch** section. Apps that can be hidden display **Installed** next to their name. Tap on the app to be hidden

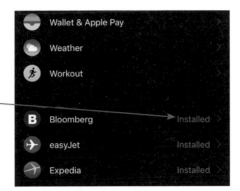

2 If the **Show App on Apple Watch** button is **On**, the app will be displayed on the Apple Watch

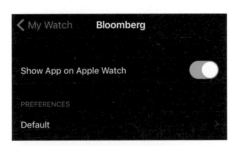

3 Drag the **Show App on Apple Watch** button to **Off**

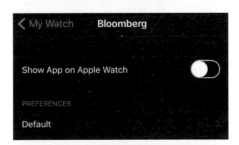

4 The app is hidden from the Apple Watch (the Installed title is no longer displayed)

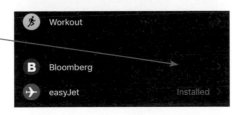

Apps are added to the Apple Watch by downloading them from the App Store on your iPhone and then syncing them with your Apple Watch (**Watch App > My Watch > General > drag Automatic App Install to On**).

To display an app that has been hidden, access it as in Step 1 and drag the **Show App on Apple Watch** button to **On**.

To delete an app, press on it gently on the Apple Watch Home screen and tap on the cross on it.

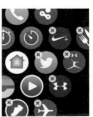

Apple Watch Straps

One of the innovations of the Apple Watch is that different straps can be used with the same watch case. For instance, you could use a sports band while monitoring your daily activity and a more sophisticated Milanese Loop when going out in the evening. Straps can quickly be removed and attached on the Apple Watch:

Hot tip

The strap can be slid either left or right to remove it.

Don't forget

The full range of straps for the Apple Watch can be viewed on the Apple website at **www.apple.com**

1 To remove the strap, press this button on the back of the Apple Watch

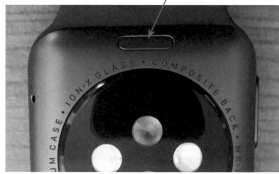

2 Slide the strap out to remove it

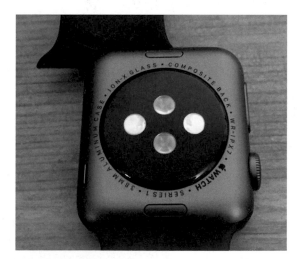

3 Slide the strap back in to attach it (the button does not have to pressed before attaching a strap)

6

More About the Apple Watch

This chapter looks at the Apple Watch in more detail, and covers some of its general uses, which make it much more than just a health and fitness band. Customizing the Watch Face is looked at, as are other functions including working with text messages and using maps to get directions.

Adding Watch Faces

Being able to use numerous Watch Faces is one of the features of the Apple Watch, and you can choose different Watch Faces to suit your mood or your current activity. Watch Faces can be changed and customized on the Apple Watch itself, and it is also possible to add new Watch Faces from the Watch app on your iPhone. To do this:

1   Tap on the **Watch** app on your iPhone

2   Tap on the **Face Gallery** button on the bottom toolbar of the Watch app

3   The different Watch Faces are displayed in their relevant main categories, e.g. Activity, Utility, Modular etc. Scroll down the page to view all of the categories

Several Watch Faces contain Complications, which are icons displaying information about items such as weather forecasts, date, World Clock and activity. Complications can be customized within Watch Faces to display different types of information. See pages 114-115 for more information about customizing Watch Faces.

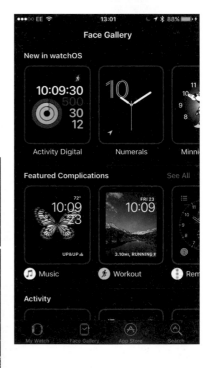

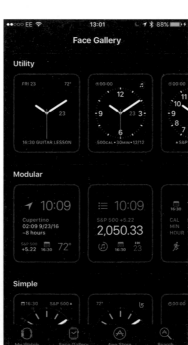

4 Tap on a Watch Face to view its details

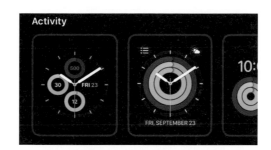

5 Details about the new Watch Face are displayed. Each face can be customized before it is added, in terms of color scheme and style

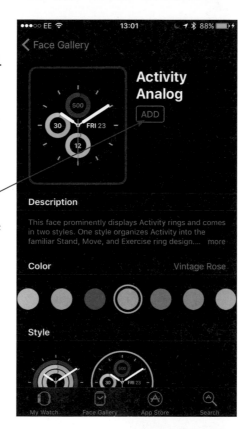

6 Tap on the **Add** button to add the Watch Face to the Apple Watch

Hot tip

Scroll down to the bottom of the screen in Step 5 to view any Complications that are included with the Watch Face, and their position, e.g. top left, top right, top, or bottom.

113

7 When a new Watch Face is added, it becomes the default one on the Apple Watch, i.e. the one that is visible from the **Clock** app

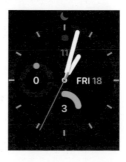

Customizing Watch Faces

Watch Faces can be customized on the Apple Watch, to change their appearance and functionality. To do this:

1 Press on the current Watch Face until the Apple Watch vibrates

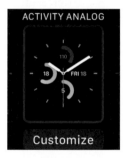

Hot tip

A number of Watch Faces contain details from the Activity app (the three colored rings) so that you can view your exercising details on the Watch Face. Tap on one of the Activity items to view the full details via the Activity app on your Apple Watch.

2 The customization mode is accessed. This contains all of the currently available Watch Faces and options for customizing them

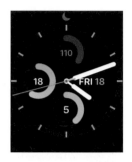

3 Swipe left and right to view all of the available Watch Faces

4 Access the required Watch Face and tap on the **Customize** button

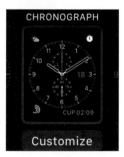

Hot tip

Press the Digital Crown to return to the current Watch Face from the screens in Steps 2 and 3.

5 Each Watch Face has its own customization options. Scroll with the Digital Crown to change the highlighted items

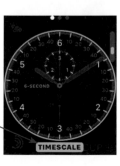

6 Swipe left and right to access different customization options. Tap on an item to select it, and use the Digital Crown to scroll through the options

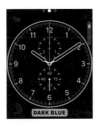 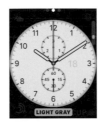

7 Small, editable items on the Watch Face are known as Complications, and can be edited by tapping on them and scrolling with the Digital Crown. This includes items such as date format and options for the Workout app, Activity app and also the World Clock

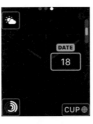 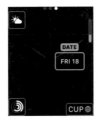

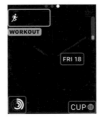 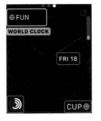

The items highlighted green are the ones that can be customized. Tap on other areas and icons to see if they can be customized too.

115

8 Once the customization has been completed, press on the Digital Crown to return to the Watch Face. The customization changes will be displayed

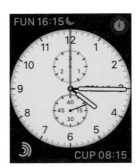

Using Siri

Siri is Apple's digital voice assistant that was first introduced on the iPhone and is now available on other Apple devices including Mac computers, iPads and the Apple Watch. On the Apple Watch the functionality is more limited since it does not have access to the web, but it can display a range of items and information. To use Siri on the Apple Watch:

Beware

On the iPhone, Hey Siri has to be trained to recognize your specific voice. However, on the Apple Watch it can be used without setting it up for a specific voice. This also means that anyone can access Siri by saying "Hey Siri".

1 Press and hold on the Digital Crown to access Siri, ready for a voice query, or

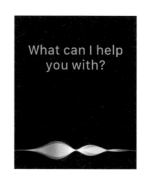

2 Open the **Settings** app

3 Tap on the **General** button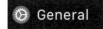

4 Tap on the **Siri** button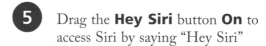

5 Drag the **Hey Siri** button **On** to access Siri by saying "Hey Siri"

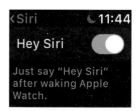

Don't forget

Hey Siri works independently from Siri on your iPhone, and it does not need to be activated on the iPhone in order to work on the Apple Watch.

6 From the Hey Siri panel, queries can be made to Siri in the same way as in Step 1, by speaking the query that you have, such as "Show my heart rate"

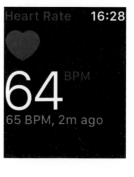

Options for Siri queries

Displaying activity information. Details from the Activity app can be accessed from Siri, so that you can view your daily targets.

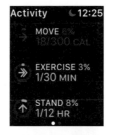

Opening apps. Siri can be used to open specific apps by saying "Open...".

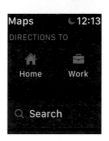

Siri can also be used for setting reminders for specific time periods, by saying "Set reminder for 15 minutes". Siri will then ask you for a subject for the reminder and play an alert at the required time.

Showing messages. You can view your latest messages via Siri by saying "Show messages". It is also possible to send messages with the Messages app by asking Siri to "Send message to X" and then speaking the text of the message.

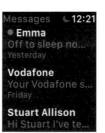

Showing sports results. Siri can display some sports results on the Apple Watch, although for others it may direct you to view them on your iPhone.

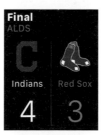

Working with iPhone. For some queries, such as viewing websites, the results have to be accessed from your iPhone, and Siri will alert you to this. Tap on the **Continue on iPhone** button to view the results.

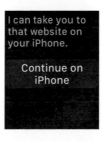

Working with Messages

Used in conjunction with your iPhone, you can receive, reply to and create messages from your Apple Watch. To reply to messages received on your Apple Watch:

1 Ensure Bluetooth is turned **On** for the iPhone

2 Tap on the **Messages** app on the Apple Watch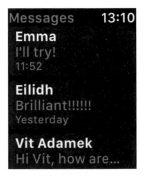

3 The latest messages are displayed. These include those that have been sent or received (from your iPhone or your Apple Watch). Tap on a message to reply to it

Messages from the Apple Watch are sent via the paired iPhone. If it is an iMessage to another iPhone/iPad user, the message bubbles will be blue; if it is to a non-Apple device, the message will be an SMS one and the message bubbles will be green.

4 The message is displayed, with reply options. Tap on the microphone button to speak a reply

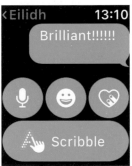

5 Create the spoken reply and tap on the **Send** button

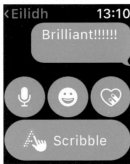

6 Tap on this button to send an emoji reply. Swipe up or down to access the available range of emojis

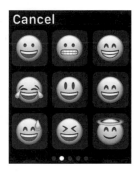

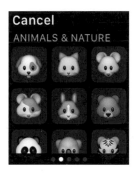

7 Tap on this button to send a Digital Touch image (which are colorful animated effects)

8 Tap on the **Scribble** button to write a message with your finger or create a drawing

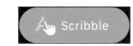

9 Scroll down the screen and tap on one of the template replies

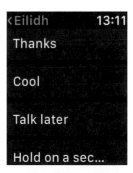

10 Press on the text window in Step 4 to access a panel with options to **Reply** to a message, view its **Details**, **Send Location** so the other person can see where you are, or **Choose Language** for using with Messages

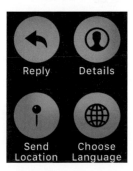

Hot tip

The press required in Step 1 is known as **Force Touch**, which is a firm press until you receive Haptic feedback (a small vibration) and the required screen appears.

...cont'd

Creating messages

To create messages on the Apple Watch:

1 Open the Messages app, press firmly on the Home screen and tap on the **New Message** button

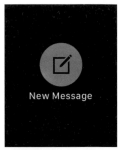

2 Tap on the **Add Contact** field

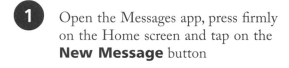

3 Select a contact from recent contacts at the bottom of the screen, or tap on this button to access your address book and select a contact here

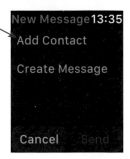

4 Create the new message with the same options as replying to a message (see pages 118-119), and tap on the **Send** button

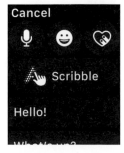

Viewing Notifications

The Apple Watch can display notifications and alerts from a range of apps. To use notifications:

1 To enable notifications for specific apps, tap on the **Watch** app on the iPhone

2 Tap on the **Notifications** button

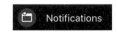

3 Drag the **Notifications Indicator** button to **On** to display a red dot at the top of the Apple Watch Face when there is a new notification

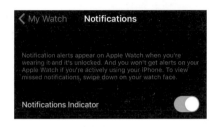

4 Tap on a specific app in the **Notifications** section to apply its settings

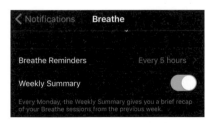

5 Notification alerts appear on the Apple Watch and can also be viewed by dragging down from the top of the Watch Face. Tap on a notification to view its details

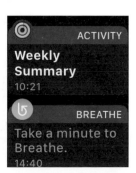

Beware

Notification alerts do not appear on the Apple Watch if the iPhone is being used.

Don't forget

The red notification indicator appears above the current Watch Face, but not on other screens.

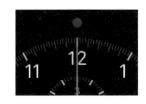

Using Maps

The Maps app on the Apple Watch can be used to show directions to locations, and display nearby facilities including restaurants, shops and cinemas. To use the Maps app:

Beware

The Home and Work addresses have to be entered in the Contacts app on your iPhone in order for the Maps app on the Apple Watch to be able to give directions to them.

1 Tap on the **Maps** icon on the Home screen

2 Tap on either **Home** or **Work** to view directions to these locations

3 Scroll down the page to view the other options

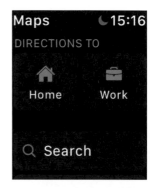

4 Tap on the **Search** button to find locations (tap on the **My Location** button to view your current location, or the **Nearby** button to view a range of facilities in the vicinity)

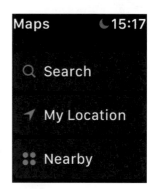

5 Tap on the **Dictation** button to dictate a location for which you want directions to, the **Favorites** button to view favorite locations (that have been added with the Maps app on the iPhone), or tap on one of the **Recents** items, which includes recent searches using the Maps app

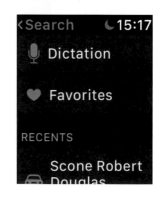

6 Tap on the required method of transport, i.e. walking, driving or transit (if transit is available)

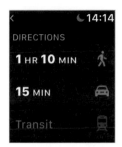

7 Once a location and mode of transport has been selected, tap on the **Start** button to get directions

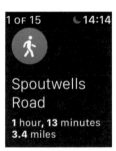

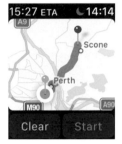

8 The Maps app on your Apple Watch displays a textual description of the route – scroll down the screen to see the whole route

Hot tip

When the **End** button in Step 9 is tapped, the route is also dismissed on the Apple Watch, and you return to the Maps app Home screen.

9 The Maps app on your iPhone opens and displays the same route, including a step-by-step process as you follow the route. Tap on the **End** button to finish following the route

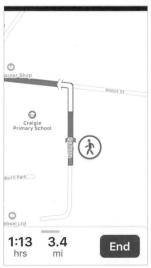

Finding Nearby Locations

The Maps app on the Apple Watch can also be used to view useful facilities relative to your own current location. To do this:

1 Tap on the **Maps** icon on the Home screen

2 Scroll down the screen and tap on the **Nearby** button

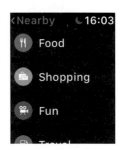

3 Tap on one of the main topics (these include **Food**, **Shopping**, **Fun** and **Travel**)

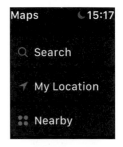

4 Tap on one of the sub-topics

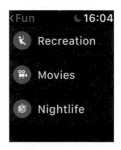

5 The relevant nearby items are listed. Tap on one to view its details

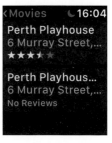

Hot tip

Tap on one of the items in Step 5 to view directions to it.

Taking Photos

Although the Apple Watch does not have its own camera, it can be used as an effective remote control for taking photos with the Camera app on your iPhone. This means that the iPhone can be situated in a different place from the Apple Watch when a photo is captured (as long as it is in range to maintain the Bluetooth connections – approximately 20 meters). To take photos using the Apple Watch and the iPhone:

125

1 Tap on the **Camera** icon on the Apple Watch's Home screen

2 The Camera app on the iPhone opens and the image is displayed on the Camera app on the Apple Watch

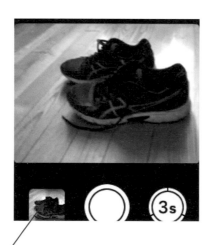

3 Tap on the shutter button on the Camera app on the Apple Watch to capture the image that is being viewed on the iPhone

4 Tap here to view the image in the **Photos** app on the Apple Watch, or open the Photos app on the Apple Watch to view all images that have been captured

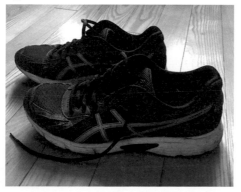

Ask a friend or family member to hold your iPhone when you are taking a photo with the Apple Watch, as it is difficult to position while using both hands to operate the Apple Watch.

To capture a screenshot (an image of what is on the screen) on the Apple Watch, hold down the Side button and press and release the Digital Crown. The image will be available in the Photos app on your iPhone. To enable screenshots, ensure that the **Enable Screenshots** options in the **Watch** app (**My Watch** > **General**) is **On**.

Beware

Only one album can be synced at a time between the iPhone and the Apple Watch.

Hot tip

Photos in the Photos app on the Apple Watch can be used to create custom Watch Faces. To do this, tap on a photo in Step 7 to view it at full size. Press on the photo and tap on the **Create Watch Face** button. The Watch Face is added to the range of available Watch Faces, and it becomes the current Watch Face.

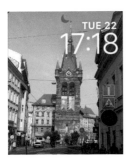

Viewing Photos

The Photos app on the Apple Watch can be used to view photos that have been taken with the Camera app on the Apple Watch, via the iPhone, and also display photos from the Photos app on the iPhone. To do this, the required albums have to be synced:

1 On the iPhone, access the **Watch** app and tap on the **My Watch** button on the bottom toolbar

2 Swipe down the screen and tap on the **Photos** button

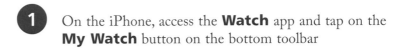

3 Tap on the **Custom** button

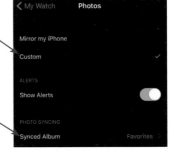

4 Tap on the **Synced Album** button

5 Tap on the album you want to sync on your Apple Watch, so that an orange tick appears next to it

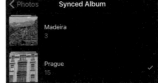

6 Tap on the **Photos** app on the Apple Watch

7 The photos from the synced album are displayed. Tap on one to view it at full size

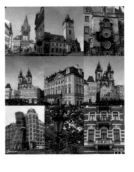

Playing Music

The Music app on the Apple Watch can be used to control the music on your iPhone, so that you do not always have to access it to play music. To do this:

1 Tap on the **Music** icon on the Apple Watch Home screen

2 Select a location from which you want to play music

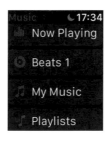

3 Tap on an item to select it, or scroll down the screen to select a category

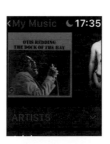

4 Tap on a track or an album to play it

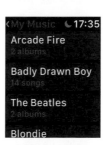

5 The song plays on your iPhone and the currently playing item is displayed on the Apple Watch

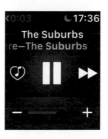

Hot tip

When playing music you can also select to play it directly from the Apple Watch, rather than on the iPhone. However, to do this you need a Bluetooth headset that is paired with the Apple Watch, using the Bluetooth option in the Settings app on the Apple Watch.

Using Apple Pay

Apple Pay is Apple's contactless payment system, first introduced with the iPhone. It works by adding credit or debit cards to the Wallet & Apple Pay app on either your Apple Watch or your iPhone, which are then authorized by the appropriate bank, and can then be used for contactless payment in participating retail outlets and websites. Apple Pay is now also available on the Apple Watch, for cards added there or on the iPhone. To set up and use Apple Pay on the Apple Watch:

Don't forget

If a debit or credit card has been added to an iPhone, it can then be added to the Apple Watch with the **Add** button in Step 3. If a new card is added with the Watch app, this will require the full process for adding and authorizing a new card for use with Apple Pay.

1 On the iPhone, tap on the **Watch** app and tap on the **My Watch** button on the bottom toolbar

2 Swipe down the screen and tap on the **Wallet & Apple Pay** button

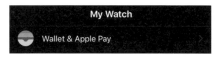

3 Tap on the **Add Credit or Debit Card** button to add a card via the iPhone, or, if one has already been added, tap on the **Add** button next to an existing card

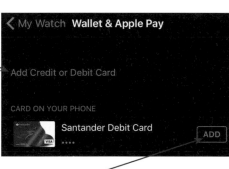

4 The card number will be displayed. Add the **Security Code** and tap on the **Next** button

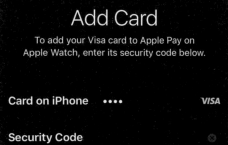

5 Select a method by which you want to verify the card (text message or phone call) and tap on the **Next** button

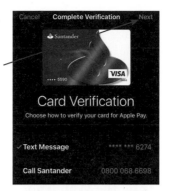

6 Enter the verification code and tap on the **Next** button

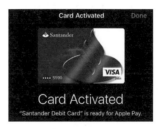

7 A confirmation screen appears once the card has been added and authorized. Tap on the **Done** button to complete the registration process

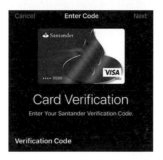

8 Tap on the **Wallet & Apple Pay** button on the Apple Watch Home screen

9 The available cards are displayed. When you have bought something and are in range of the contactless payment terminal, hold the Apple Watch near to the terminal, then **Double-click** the **Side button** to pay for an item with Apple Pay

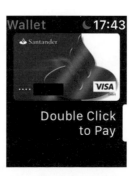

When you use Apple Pay on your Apple Watch to pay for something in a retail outlet for the first time, try to do so when there is not a long queue behind you, just so that you have plenty of time to complete the process.

Finding a Lost Apple Watch

Although the Apple Watch will probably be worn for most of the time, there will always be occasions when you have to take it off your wrist. This leads to the possibility that it could get lost or mislaid. If this happens, or worse, it is stolen, it is possible to try to locate a missing Apple Watch and display it on an online map. If required, it can also be locked or erased remotely, if you are concerned that its contents may be compromised. A missing Apple Watch can be found with either the Watch app on the iPhone or the Find iPhone app on the iPhone.

Using the Watch app
To find a lost or missing Apple Watch using the Watch app:

Don't forget

To use the Find My Apple Watch option, an Apple ID is required. This is a username (usually an email address) and a password that can be used to access a range of Apple's online services, including iTunes, App Store, iBooks, iMessages, FaceTime and iCloud, the online storage and backup service. An Apple ID can be created when you first access one of the associated services, or on the Apple website at https://appleid.apple.com/account

1 On the iPhone, tap on the **Watch** app and tap on the **My Watch** button on the bottom toolbar

2 Tap on the Apple Watch name

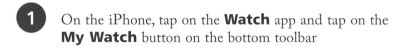
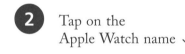

3 Tap on the **i** icon next to the Apple Watch name

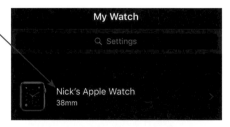

4 Tap on the **Find My Apple Watch** button

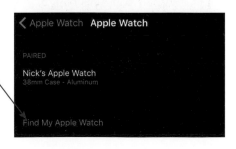
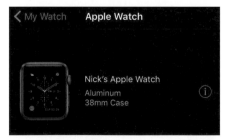

5 An Apple ID is required to use the Find My iPhone feature. Enter the required details and tap on the **Sign In...** button

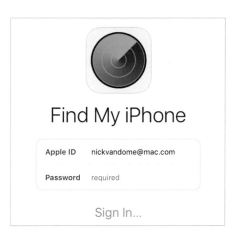

Find My iPhone

Apple ID	nickvandome@mac.com
Password	required

Sign In...

6 The missing Apple Watch is shown on a map, with a range of **Actions** on the bottom toolbar. Swipe outwards with thumb and forefinger to zoom in on the map

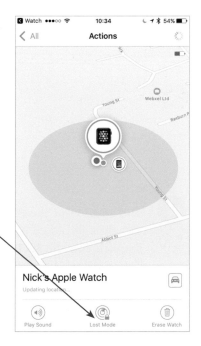

7 Tap on the **Lost Mode** button on the bottom toolbar

8 Tap on the **Turn On Lost Mode** button to activate this so that you can lock your Apple Watch remotely so that no-one else can use it (a passcode will be required to unlock it)

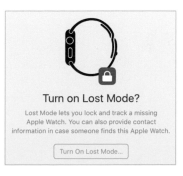

Turn on Lost Mode?

Lost Mode lets you lock and track a missing Apple Watch. You can also provide contact information in case someone finds this Apple Watch.

Turn On Lost Mode...

Beware

Tap on the **Erase Watch** button in Step 6 to delete all settings and content from the Apple Watch. Only do this if you are concerned that the Apple Watch has fallen into the wrong hands. (Data that has been synced to the iPhone will be retained.)

131

Hot tip

Tap on the **Play Sound** button in Step 6 to play a sound from the Apple Watch. This is a good option if the Apple Watch is missing in the home or office. Tap on the **Dismiss** button on the Apple Watch once you have found it.

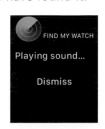

FIND MY WATCH

Playing sound...

Dismiss

...cont'd

Using the Find iPhone app

The Find iPhone app on your iPhone can also be used to find a missing Apple Watch (and other Apple devices). To do this:

A missing Apple Watch can also be located from the iCloud website. This is Apple's online storage and backup service that can also be used to share content between compatible devices. An iCloud account can be created when you set up a new iPhone or iPad, or when a new Apple ID is created. The iCloud website at **www.icloud.com** can then be used to access your iCloud content, including the **Find iPhone** option for locating missing devices such as the Apple Watch.

The Find iPhone service covers all compatible devices, including iPads, Mac computers and the Apple Watch, not just the iPhone.

1 On the iPhone, tap on the **Find iPhone** app

2 **Sign In** with your Apple ID, as on page 131

3 All of the compatible Apple devices are listed. Tap on the name of your Apple Watch

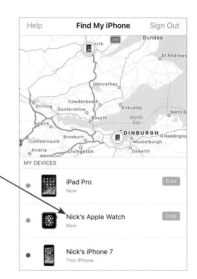

4 The location of the Apple Watch is displayed on a map. Tap on the **Actions** button on the bottom toolbar to access the same actions for working with a missing or lost Apple Watch, as in Step 6 on page 131

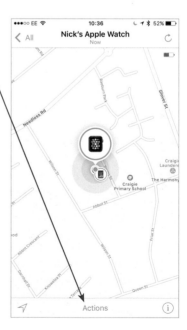

7

Using the Activity App

The Activity app is one of the main elements on the Apple Watch and can be used to record your daily fitness activities. This chapter details using the app and viewing the daily goals.

About the Activity App

Health and fitness is one of the main uses for the Apple Watch, and one of the items that is fundamental to this is the Activity app. There are complementary versions on both the Apple Watch and the iPhone, and they communicate fully with each other. This means that you can collect your health and fitness data on your Apple Watch and view a summary of it there, and then view a fuller analysis of the data on your iPhone.

The Activity app is used to measure three separate fitness metrics:

- **Stand**. This is used to measure how many times that you stand and move for at least one minute within an hour.

- **Move**. This is used to measure how many active calories you burn each day (this is calculated as calories over the standard number of calories burned when you are inactive).

- **Exercise**. This measures the amount of exercise that you take each day, based on activity at a rate over that of a brisk walk.

Setting up the Activity app

The Activity app can be set up during the process of pairing the Apple Watch and the iPhone (see page 88). This sets the required targets for each goal. To do this during the pairing process on the iPhone:

To achieve the Stand goal each hour, you have to move around too, rather than just standing still for a period of time.

1 In the Activity setup screen, tap on the **Set up Activity** button

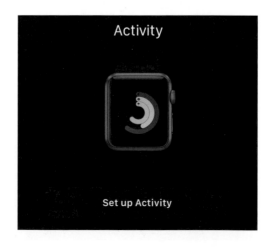

134

2 Enter personal details, including weight and height, which will be used by the Activity app to help monitor your goals. Tap on the **Continue** button

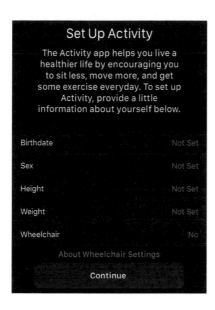

3 Set a figure for the number of calories for the Move goal and tap on the **Set Move Goal** button

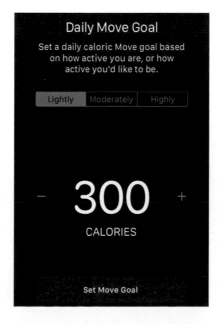

The Move goal is the only one that can be edited: the Exercise and Stand goals cannot be changed. See page 139 for details about changing the Move goal.

...cont'd

Activity app on the Apple Watch

To use the Activity app on the Apple Watch:

1 Tap on the **Activity** app on the Home screen

2 Swipe to the left to move through the introductory screen, and then tap on the **Get Started** button

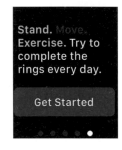

Stand. Move. Exercise. Try to complete the rings every day.

Get Started

3 The three rings indicate the progress towards each of the daily goals

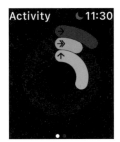

Activity 11:30

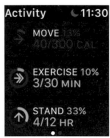

Activity 11:30

MOVE 13%
40/300 CAL

EXERCISE 10%
3/30 MIN

STAND 33%
4/12 HR

4 Scroll down the screen to view the progress of the daily goals

5 Scroll down the screen to view the daily goals in graph format, displayed per hour

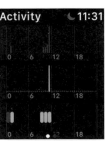

Activity 11:31

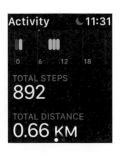

Activity 11:31

TOTAL STEPS
892

TOTAL DISTANCE
0.66 KM

6 Scroll down the screen to view the number of steps that have been taken and the distance covered

Don't forget

Settings for the Activity app can be applied using the Watch app on the iPhone, see page 138.

Don't forget

The objective for the Activity app is to complete or surpass the three rings each day.

Activity app on the iPhone

The Activity app is also available on the iPhone, and this shows the same details as on the Apple Watch but in a larger and more in-depth display. To view this:

1 Tap on the **Activity** app on the Home screen

2 The three rings indicate the progress towards each of the daily goals (as on the Apple Watch)

3 Scroll down the screen to view graphs for the daily goals

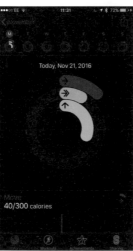

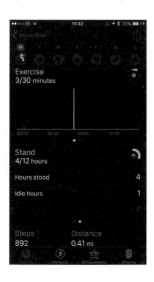

4 Swipe to the left on a panel to view the details of each graph

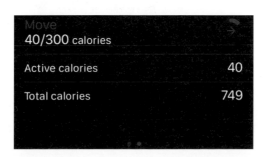

The Activity app only appears on the iPhone once it has been paired with the Apple Watch.

Activity data cannot be recorded in the Activity app on the iPhone; it has to be synced from the Apple Watch.

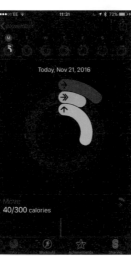
Bluetooth has to be turned **On** on the iPhone (**Settings** > **Bluetooth**) in order for the Activity app to sync with the version on the Apple Watch.

Tap on a date on the top toolbar to view the data for that date. Tap on the month name to see the monthly view. The current day is highlighted red in month view.

Activity App Settings

The settings for the Activity app are applied within the Watch app on the iPhone. To do this:

1 Tap on the **Watch** app on the iPhone Home screen

2 Tap on the **My Watch** button on the bottom toolbar

3 Swipe down the screen and tap on the **Activity** button

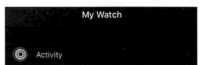

4 Drag the buttons **On** or **Off** for the Activity app Settings. These include: muting reminders, **Stand Reminders** if you have been sitting for too long, **Progress Updates**, notifications when you reach **Goal Completions**, when you reach an **Achievements**, and a **Weekly Summary**

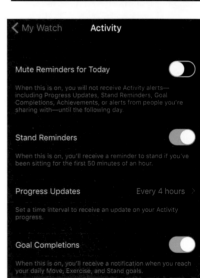

Turning the **Stand Reminders** to **On** is a good idea if you work at a desk for long periods of time. The reminder is sent after the first 50 minutes of inactivity in an hour.

If **Do Not Disturb** is **On** for the Apple Watch (**Settings** > **Do Not Disturb**), notification alerts will not be played.

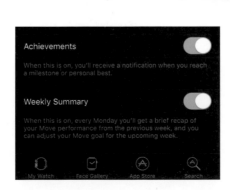

Changing Move Goals

The Move goal on the Activity app is the only one that can be edited, and this is done in the Activity app on the Apple Watch. To edit the Move goal on the Apple Watch:

1 Tap on the **Activity** app on the Home screen

2 Press on any of the Activity app's screens, e.g. the rings, details or graphs screens

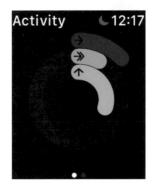

3 Tap on the **Change Move Goal** button (the **Weekly Summary** button accesses a screen where you see details of days in the previous week when you beat your Move goal, and totals for the other Activity goals – see page 140)

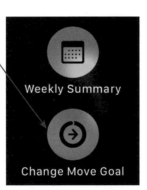

4 Enter a new move goal using the **-** or **+** buttons (or by turning the Digital Crown) and tap on the **Update** button

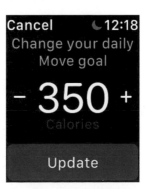

Beware

Do not set the Move goal too high, otherwise it could become dispiriting if you keep missing it. It is better to have a goal that you can achieve on a regular basis, to maintain your motivation. Increase it by small amounts if you exceed the goal on a regular basis.

Viewing Weekly Activity

The Activity app on the Apple Watch displays your daily activity for the three rings (Move, Exercise and Stand), and the task is to try to close these rings, e.g. complete the goals, each day. However, it is also possible to view a weekly summary of all of your activity. To do this:

1 On your Apple Watch, tap on the **Activity** app

2 Press on the three rings screen until it vibrates slightly and the screen in Step 3 appears

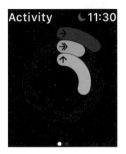

Hot tip

If notifications have been set up for the Activity app on the Apple Watch (**iPhone Watch app** > **My Watch** > **Notifications** > **Activity**), the Weekly Summary can also be accessed by swiping down from the top of the screen from any Watch Face. This is available each Monday.

3 Tap on the **Weekly Summary** button

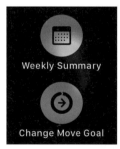

4 Scroll through the summary to view all of the details relating to your Activity rings, steps walked and distance covered

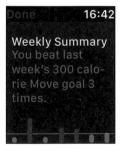

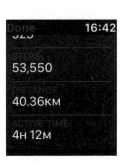

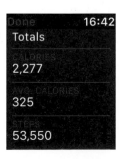

140

Standing Goals

The Stand goal on the Activity app may seem the simplest, but it can sometimes be a challenge to meet the 12 hours of standing and moving for at least one minute every hour, particularly for people with a sedentary job. However, the Apple Watch does its best to encourage you to meet your goal:

1 On your Apple Watch, tap on the **Activity** app

2 Scroll down the page to view the Stand details. A solid line indicates an hour that has been completed. A pale line indicates an hour that has only been partially completed

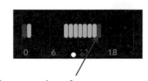

3 Open the **Watch** app on your iPhone, and under the **My Watch** section, tap on **Notifications > Activity** and drag the **Stand Reminders** button to **On**

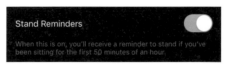

4 If you do not stand or move for the first 50 minutes of an hour, the Apple Watch will display a reminder to complete your goal

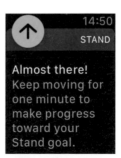

5 Once the goal has been completed after the reminder, a confirmation message appears

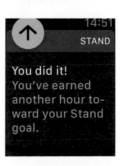

Hot tip

The number of Stand hours is also displayed in the Health app on the iPhone.

Achieving Awards

Receiving awards is a good way to keep motivated when doing health and fitness activities, and the Activity app recognizes your achievements and rewards you accordingly, with virtual awards. These are for a range of achievements, so that you are inspired to keep up with your activities. To view your achievement rewards:

Although the Activity app awards may seem a simplistic way to encourage you to do more exercise, it can be surprisingly effective when you get them, and it is a good way to monitor your progress.

1 On your iPhone, tap on the **Activity** app

2 Tap on the **Achievements** button on the bottom toolbar

3 The available achievement rewards are listed on the screen. The ones in color are the ones that have been obtained at least once (some awards can be achieved on several occasions)

Awards are also given for activity performed with the Workout app (see Chapter Eight).

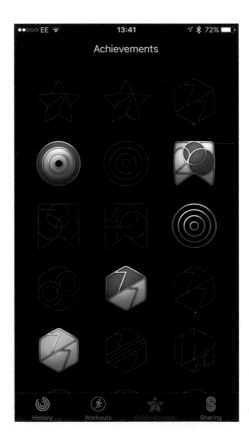

4 Tap on an award icon to view its details and see what the award is given for

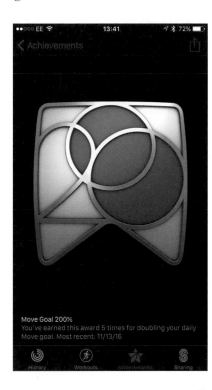

Some of the criteria for which awards are given are: doubling, tripling or quadrupling your daily Move goal; new Move record; eight consecutive days of achieving your Move goal; reaching your Move goal for an entire week; reaching your daily Exercise goal for an entire week (from Monday to Sunday); reaching your daily Stand goal for an entire week; reaching all of your Activity ring goals for an entire week; reaching your Move goals for an entire month; achieving your Move goal 100, 365, 500 and 1000 times.

5 Tap on the **History** button on the bottom toolbar

6 Select a specific date, and swipe to the bottom of the page to view any rewards that have been achieved on that day

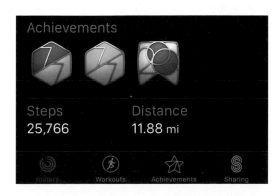

Every time an award is achieved, a blue dot appears underneath it.

Sharing Activities

Sharing information from the Activity app is a good way to include family and friends in your exercise activities: it can also encourage mutual support, even if it is by competing with other people to see who can get the best results. To share your Activity app information:

1 On your iPhone, tap on the **Activity** app

2 Tap on the **Sharing** button on the bottom toolbar

3 Tap on the **Get Started** button to invite people to participate

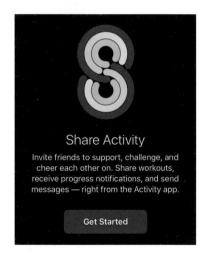

Share Activity

Invite friends to support, challenge, and cheer each other on. Share workouts, receive progress notifications, and send messages — right from the Activity app.

Get Started

4 Tap on the **+** button in the **Activity Sharing** window to invite other people to share information from the Activity app

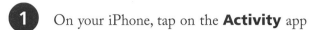
Activity Sharing +

5 Enter the details for the people with whom you want to share information

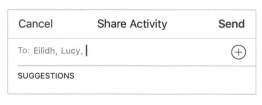

Cancel	Share Activity	Send
To: Eilidh, Lucy,		⊕
SUGGESTIONS		

from the Activity app, and tap on the **Send** button

Beware

If you want to share information from the Activity app, the other person has to have an Apple Watch too.

144

Obtaining More Activity Apps

The Activity app on the Apple Watch and iPhone is an excellent method of recording and storing information from your exercising activities. However, there are also other useful activity and workout apps that can be downloaded from the App Store.

1 Tap on the **Watch** app on the iPhone Home screen

2 Tap on the **App Store** button on the bottom toolbar

3 Apps that have Apple Watch versions, in addition to iPhone versions, are displayed

4 Tap on an app to view its details, or tap on the **See All** button to view all of the apps in that category

5 Tap on the **Search** button on the bottom toolbar to search for apps with specific keywords, e.g. Activity

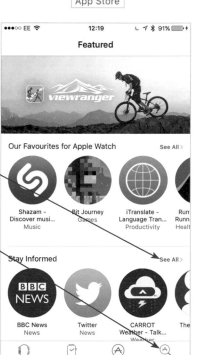

Search

6 Enter the keyword(s) and tap on one of the results to view related apps

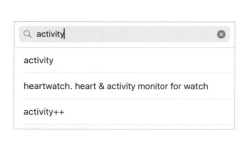

The range of apps for the Apple Watch is more limited than that for the iPhone or iPad, but there are nevertheless some very useful apps, and the range is increasing on a regular basis.

...cont'd

Don't forget

If an app is free, it will display the Get button; if it is paid-for it will display its price.

Hot tip

To ensure the app is automatically added to the Apple Watch from the iPhone, select **Watch app** > **My Watch** > **General** and drag **Automatic App Install** to **On**.

Beware

Some apps have in-app purchases, whereby the initial app is free, but additional items have to be bought once you are using the app, if you want to increase its functionality.

7 Review the apps by tapping on them to see their details. Tap on the **Get** (or price) button to obtain an app

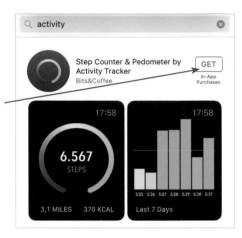

8 Tap on the **Install** button to start downloading the app

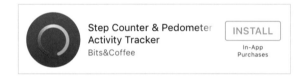

9 The app icon appears on the iPhone Home screen

10 The app icon also appears on the Apple Watch Home screen

11 Apple Watch apps can also be downloaded directly from the App Store on your iPhone. Look for the **Offers Apple Watch App** text next to an app, and tap on the Get (or price) button to download it in the same way as above

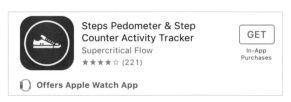

8 Using the Workout App

The Workout app is another Apple Watch app, which can be used to record specific exercise workouts. This chapter shows how to use the app, and view workout data.

About the Workout App

While the Activity app is excellent for meeting the needs of recording your daily activity, the Workout app takes this a step further by being able to record specific periods of activity, such as running or gym work. This can then be stored in the Activity app on the iPhone, so that you can see details about all of your activities in one place. To start using the Workout app:

Don't forget

The Workout app is only on the Apple Watch, and there is no comparable version on the iPhone. However, the workout details appear in the Activity app and the Health app.

148

Don't forget

The available workouts in the Workout app are: Outdoor Walk, Outdoor Run, Outdoor Cycle, Indoor Walk, Indoor Run, Indoor Cycle, Elliptical, Rower, Stair Stepper and Other, for workouts that do not fit any of the other options.

1 Tap on the **Workout** app icon on the Apple Watch's Home screen

2 The types of available workouts are listed. Scroll down the page to view all of the options, including **Other**, if your workout does not fit any of the options

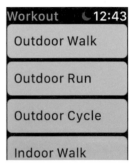

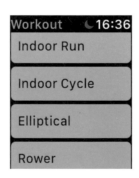
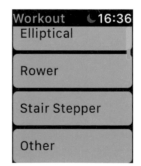

3 For some types of workout you will be prompted to take your iPhone with you during the first 20 minutes, so that the Apple Watch can record all elements of your workout accurately (this only has to be done once)

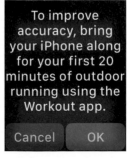

To improve accuracy, bring your iPhone along for your first 20 minutes of outdoor running using the Workout app.

Cancel   OK

...cont'd

4 Tap on the type of workout that you want to perform, and enter a goal for the number of calories that you want to burn (these are active calories which are those burned in excess of those burned during your normal resting rate)

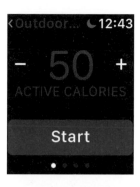

Use the **+** or **-** buttons to enter the figures for Steps 4, 5 and 6, or turn the Digital Crown to change the figures.

5 Swipe to the left and enter the duration that you want the workout to last for

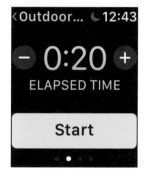

Press and hold on the Active Calories option in Step 4 to select whether this displays as **Active Calories** or **Kilojoules**.

6 Swipe to the left and enter the required distance for the workout (if applicable)

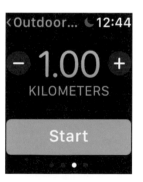

All workouts have options for Active Calories and Elapsed Time, but they only have Kilometers if applicable, e.g. for a walk, run or cycle.

7 Swipe to the left and **Start** the workout from the **Open** panel, to have no goal for the workout

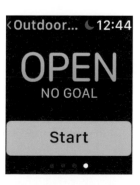

Press and hold on the Kilometers option in Step 6 to select whether this displays as **Kilometers** or **Miles**.

Starting a Workout

After the criteria have been set, as on page 149, you can start your workout:

as on page 149

150

Hot tip

Turn the Digital Crown to highlight different elements of the workout readout, e.g. the time, active calories, heart rate or distance.

1 From any of the screens on page 149, tap on the **Start** button to begin a workout

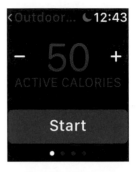

2 The Apple Watch displays a countdown to the beginning of the workout, so that you can start it as accurately as possible

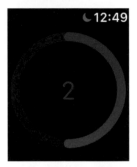

3 At the beginning of the workout, there is no data to display (except for the stopwatch starting). The app can be paused if you stop a workout and then restart it

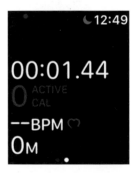

4 As the workout progresses, the workout data is displayed and changes as the workout continues. This includes your heart rate which is recorded with the **Heart Rate** app on the Apple Watch

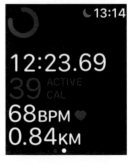

5 The Workout app notifies you when you achieve certain milestones towards the goals set for the workout

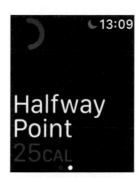

6 This circle at the top of the screen displays the progress of the workout goals

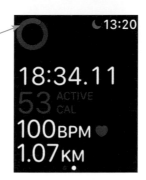

The color of the circle in the top left-hand corner of the Workout app depends on the goal from which the workout was started: if it is the Calorie goal, it will be red; if it is the Time goal, it will be yellow; and if it is the Distance goal, it will be blue.

7 Swipe to the right to access the controls for the current workout. Tap on the **Pause** button to pause the current workout. Tap on the **End** button to finish the workout. Tap on the **Lock** button to lock the screen so that it cannot be changed

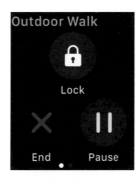

Turn the Digital Crown away from you to unlock the Apple Watch if it has been locked with the option in Step 7.

8 If a workout has been paused, tap on the **Resume** button to continue it

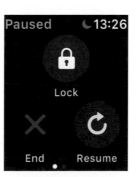

Completing a Workout

Once a workout has been completed, there is a range of data that can be viewed and analyzed, using the Workout app. To do this:

The Workout app also records the date and time at which the workout was performed.

1 The Apple Watch displays a **Summary** of the workout once it has been completed

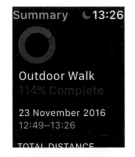

Summary ☾ 13:26

Outdoor Walk
114% Complete

23 November 2016
12:49–13:26

TOTAL DISTANCE

The total number of calories is calculated with the number of active calories plus those used at rest.

2 Scroll down the Summary page, using the Digital Crown, or by swiping. The summary includes the total distance covered (if applicable), the total time of the workout, the number of active calories used...

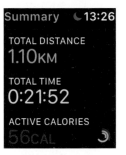

Summary ☾ 13:26

TOTAL DISTANCE
1.10KM

TOTAL TIME
0:21:52

ACTIVE CALORIES
56CAL

...the total number of calories used, the average pace of the workout (for walking, running or cycling), the average heart rate...

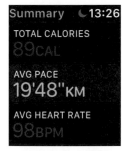

Summary ☾ 13:26

TOTAL CALORIES
89CAL

AVG PACE
19'48"KM

AVG HEART RATE
98BPM

...the elevation gained during the workout, and the weather conditions at the time

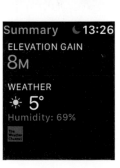

Summary ☾ 13:26

ELEVATION GAIN
8M

WEATHER
☀ 5°
Humidity: 69%

3 At the bottom of the screen, tap on options to either **Save** or **Discard** the workout

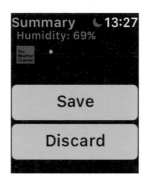

4 Once a workout has been saved the data can be viewed in the Activity app on your iPhone. A summary of the workout also appears on the Workout app. Tap on **Quick Start** to repeat the workout with the same goals as the initial one

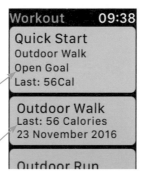

Hot tip

The item shown under **Last** for the most recent workout is the one from which the workout was started, e.g. calories, time or distance.

153

5 A summary of the workout also appears under **Last** for the category of workout. Tap on this to repeat the workout, but with amended goals. By default, the Workout app increases the goals to just above what was achieved in the previous workout

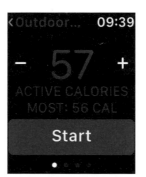

Hot tip

When you complete your first workout with the Workout app, you receive an award in the **Achievements** section of the Activity app on your iPhone.

6 Accept the new suggested goals, or apply new ones in the same way as for settings them in the first place. Tap on the **Start** button to perform the workout with the new goals

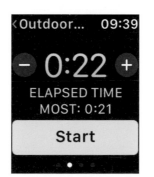

Viewing Workout Details

Due to its size, the Apple Watch is not ideal for viewing in-depth details about workouts. Instead, the Activity app on the iPhone, and also the Health app, can be used to view and analyze your workout activity. To do this:

1 Tap on the **Activity** app on the iPhone Home screen

2 Tap on the **Workouts** button on the bottom toolbar

Hot tip

Tap on the **Share** button to share the workout details with family and friends, via a text message, email or social media sites.

3 Tap on a workout to view its details

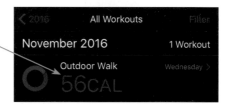

4 The workout screen shows the same information as on the Apple Watch, but the main figures can all be viewed on the same screen. Swipe down the screen to view more details

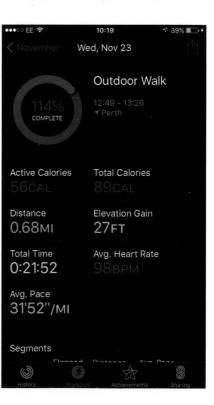

5 The Activity app also displays segments for the workout. This is determined by the app by automatically breaking up the workout into several sections

Segments			
	Elapsed Time	Distance (mi)	Avg. Pace (/mi)
01	05:47	0.28	20'37"
02	00:20	0	--'--"
03	00:37	0	--'--"
04	15:07	0.41	37'15"

Route	Weather
	☀ 42°
	Humidity: 69%

Segments are a good way to compare your progress if you do the same workout: you can view the same segments for the workout, including the times on each occasion.

6 Tap on the **Route** icon to view the route of the workout on a map. Tap on the date to move back to the main window

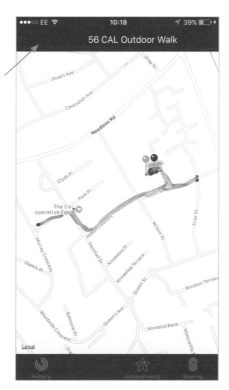

Apple Watch Series 2 has built-in GPS, so the paired iPhone does not need to be taken with it in order to map the route of a workout. However, Series 1 requires the iPhone to be taken with the Apple Watch, to provide the GPS.

...cont'd

Using the Health app to view workout data

The Health app can also display workout information, from the Apple Watch and also other sources:

If you are looking at the Health app on the same day as the workout was completed, the details will also be available from the **Today** button on the bottom toolbar.

1 Tap on the **Health** app on the iPhone Home screen

2 Tap on the **Health Data** button on the bottom toolbar

3 Tap on the **Activity** button

4 Tap on a workout to view its details

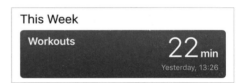

Don't forget

Use the **Day**, **Week**, **Month** and **Year** buttons at the top of the screen in Step 5 to view all workout information on a graph for these time periods.

5 The Workouts screen displays all workout information that the Health app has collated, from a variety of sources. Tap on the **Show All Data** button to view specific details

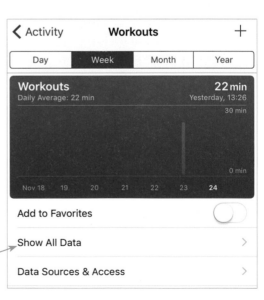

6 Details of all recorded workouts are displayed. Tap on ones with the Apple Watch icon next to them to view their details

7 The recorded details are displayed, including the type of workout, the date and time of the workout, the source, and the **Workout Samples** (at the bottom of the screen)

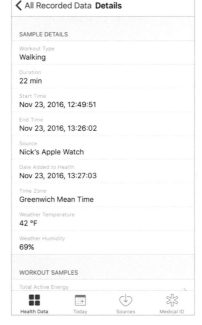

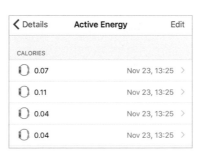

8 Tap on one of the Workout Samples options to view the points at which the data was collected

Don't forget

The Health app is a good option for collating workout information, as it shows data from multiple sources, as does the Activity app, i.e. if you have performed a workout with a third-party workout app from the App Store.

Workout App Settings

The items that appear on the Workout app on the Apple Watch (during a workout), and the order in which they appear, can be customized within the Activity app on the iPhone. To do this:

1 Tap on the **Activity** app on the iPhone Home screen

2 Tap on the **My Watch** button on the bottom toolbar

3 Scroll down the page and tap on the **Workout** button

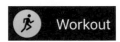

4 Tap on the **Workout View** button

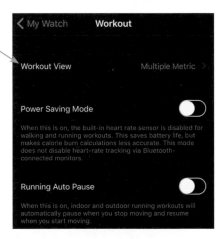

The other two options in Step 4 are for **Power Saving Mode** and **Running Auto Pause**. Power Saving Mode can be turned **On** to save battery power, but this means the heart rate sensor is disabled, so the calculations for calories burned may be less accurate. Running Auto Pause can be turned **On** so that running workouts will automatically pause when you stop moving, and resume when you start again.

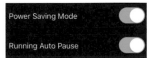

5 Tap on the **Multiple Metric** button to edit the range of metrics that appear on the Apple Watch during a workout

6 Tap on one of the **Workouts** to view and edit its metrics

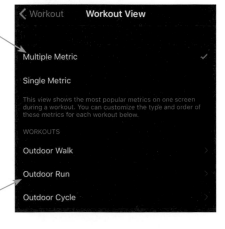

...cont'd

7 The metrics that are included, and their order, are shown at the top of the screen. Items that are not included, but available, are shown at the bottom of the screen, under **Do Not Include**

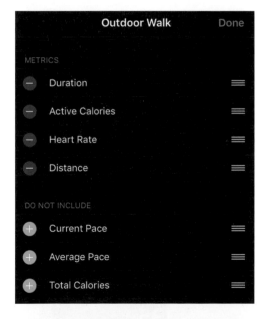

The metrics in Step 7 are those that appear on the Apple Watch Face while a workout is in progress; they are not the goals that are set before the workout starts.

159

8 Tap on the **Edit** button to enable items to be added or removed, and change the order in which they appear

9 Tap on the red circle next to an item and tap on the **Remove** button

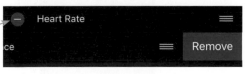

...cont'd

10 Items that have been removed appear under the **Do Not Include** heading. Tap on a green circle to add an item from here

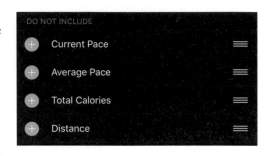

11 Press on this button and drag to change the order of the metrics

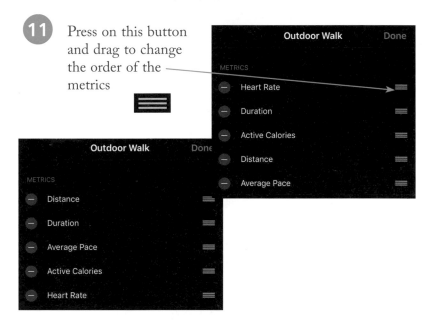

Tap on the **Done** button to apply editing changes to the metrics.

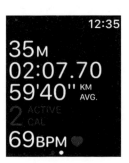

12 The order of the metrics in Step 11 is replicated on the Apple Watch during a workout

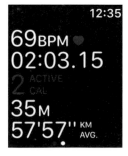

Workout Achievements

As with the three goals on the Activity app, there are achievement awards that can be collected for workouts with the Workout app, to keep you encouraged and motivated. To view these:

1 Tap on the **Activity** app on the iPhone Home screen

2 Tap on the **Achievements** button on the bottom toolbar

3 There is an award for the first time you complete a workout

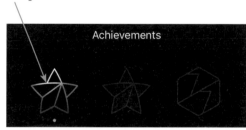

There are only three available awards for activities related to the Workout app. There are 16 related to activities for the Activities app.

4 There is an award for every time you beat your record of most calories burned, after completing at least five workouts

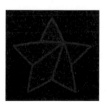

5 There is an award for when you complete seven workouts of at least 15 minutes in one week

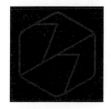

More Workout Apps

In addition to the Activity and the Workout apps on the Apple Watch, there are also numerous apps that perform workout functions that can be downloaded from the App Store. Fitness data from these apps can also be collated and viewed using the Activity app on the iPhone:

1 Tap on the **Activity** app on the iPhone Home screen

2 Tap on the **Workouts** button on the bottom toolbar

3 Workouts that have been added from other apps are denoted by the app's icon next to them

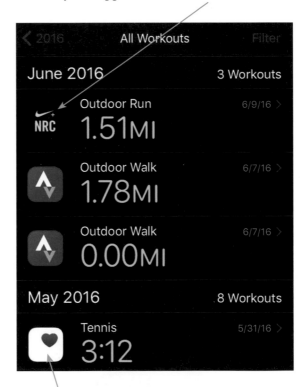

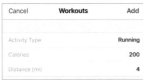

> Workout details can be added manually to the Health app. To do this, access the Workouts section within the Activity category and tap on this button ⊞ at the top of the screen. Enter the required data, and tap on the **Add** button.

Cancel	Workouts	Add
Activity Type		Running
Calories		200
Distance (mi)		4

4 Workouts that have been recorded from the Health app are also listed in the Activity app

Some of the workout and activity apps that can be downloaded to your Apple Watch and iPhone from the App Store are:

7 Minute Workout

This is an app that can be used to follow 12 quick workouts for a selection of disciplines. These include push-ups, sit-ups, jumping jacks and lunges. The workouts are split up into 30-second periods of exercise, with 10 seconds between each exercise. The workouts are designed to exercise all parts of your body.

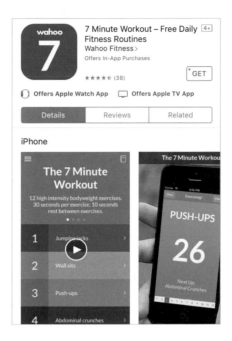

FitStar Personal Trainer

This is an app that has video routines from fitness trainers to follow, without the need to get your own personal fitness trainer. FitStar tracks your fitness progress and then adapts the exercises and routines to your current level of fitness. An active internet connection is required to view the full range of FitStar exercise videos.

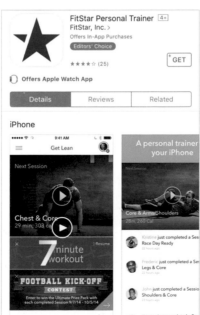

Apps can be downloaded from the **App Store** app on the iPhone, but if you do this, make sure that they say **Offers Apple Watch App** on their details, if you want to use the apps with your Apple Watch. Apps for the Apple Watch (and the iPhone) can be downloaded from the **Watch** app on the iPhone by tapping on the **Search** button on the bottom toolbar to find apps in the App Store.

163

Drink plenty of water during and after a workout, to avoid getting dehydrated.

The FitStar videos only play on the iPhone version of the app, not the Apple Watch version.

...cont'd

Zova

This is an app that comes with your own virtual reality personal trainer: Zara. She can be used to track your workout activity and give you tips and encouragement. The app can be used to track walking, running and full-body workouts. There is also a paid-for Premium version of Zova, and this can be used to create your own tailored workouts.

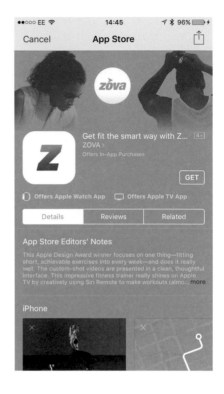

The Apple Watch version of workout apps tends to just show activity information, rather than the workouts themselves.

164

Personal Trainer by Track My Fitness

This is another app that provides video workouts, covering different time periods, fitness levels, types of workouts and equipment used. There are also workout challenges that you can take on and record for your daily, weekly and monthly activity.

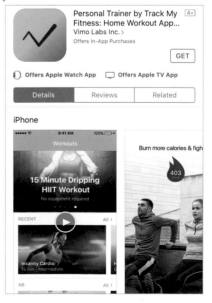

Runtastic Results

This is an app that offers a 12-week training plan, using bodyweight exercises that do not require any special equipment. It assesses your fitness and then tailors the workout routines to your own specific needs. It also has a health and nutrition guide to aid your overall health and fitness. In total, there are over 150 workout videos that can be used, all in HD. The results of each workout are available to view on your Apple Watch.

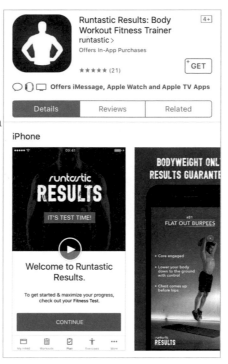

For more advanced routines, most workout apps have a premium version that has to be paid for.

Sworkit

This is another app that offers personalized video workouts, covering strength, cardio, yoga and stretching. The times of the workouts vary from five minutes to an hour, and they are conducted by a video trainer to guide you through the exercises.

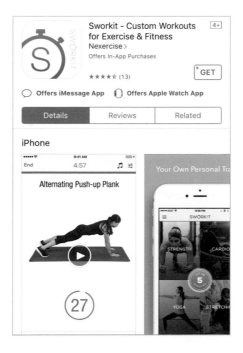

...cont'd

Workout Tracker Gym Log

This is an app for fitness, bodybuilding and workout enthusiasts. It has over 1300 exercises with descriptions and animated personal trainers. It can be used to create personal workouts, track a range of workout information, and share and compare the results with friends to create a collaborative environment.

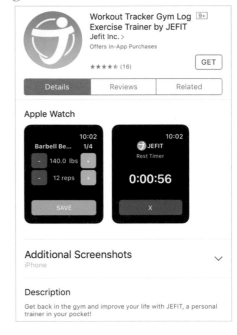

Beware

Don't undertake any workouts if you are feeling ill or have an injury: it will most likely only make things worse.

Workout Trainer

This is another virtual personal trainer app, which uses audio, photos and videos to guide you through numerous workout scenarios. You can also undertake a virtual fitness assessment and there is a 'workout for a week' challenge. It is also possible to set reminders to schedule your workouts so that you can create a weekly routine.

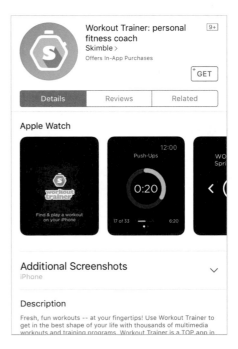

9 General Health and Wellbeing

This chapter looks at some general health and fitness issues, including taking your heart rate, maintaining a healthy diet, and some equipment for keeping fit.

Monitoring Heart Rate

The heart rate sensor and app on the Apple Watch can provide details of your heart rate, which can then be viewed in the Health app on your iPhone. This is a useful guide to your heart rate, but not a definitive indicator as to the physical condition of your heart, or your overall health. However, it is a good way to track your heart rate over a period of time, and during different levels of exercise. To monitor your heart rate:

If you have any concerns about your heart rate, or any other aspect of your health, see your doctor immediately.

Heart rate is measured as BPM – Beats Per Minute.

The Workout app on the Apple Watch can also display your heart rate during a workout.

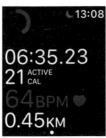

1 Tap on the **Heart Rate** app on the Home screen of the Apple Watch

2 When it is first accessed, the Heart Rate app takes a few seconds to display the heart rate

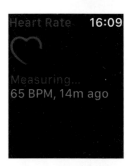

3 The current heart rate is displayed, with the previously recorded figure underneath it

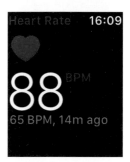

4 Measure your heart rate during different levels of exercise to see the difference and also the time it takes to revert to your normal heart rate following exercise

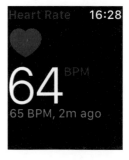

Viewing heart rate data

The Health app on the iPhone can be used to view archived heart rate data and the heart rate range for specific dates. To do this:

1 Tap on the **Health** app on the iPhone Home screen

2 Tap on the **Health Data** button on the bottom toolbar

3 Tap on the **Vitals** button

4 The most recently recorded heart rate is displayed. Tap on this button to view its details

5 The standard Health app graph is displayed, with a record of all recorded heart rates, showing the minimum and maximum limits

6 Tap on the **Show All Data** button to view all of the archived heart rate information

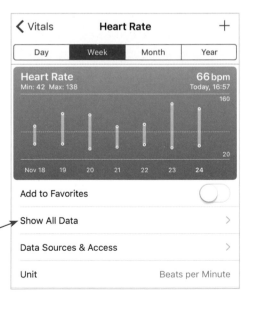

The Health app obtains heart rate data automatically from the Heart Rate app on the Apple Watch, providing that the iPhone and Apple Watch have been paired and the iPhone has Bluetooth On.

The heart rate data can also be accessed from the **Today** button on the bottom toolbar of the Health app, providing that heart rate data has been recorded during the current day.

169

...cont'd

7 The daily heart rate data is displayed, showing the range of the lowest and highest heart rate for each day

⟨ Heart Rate **All Recorded Data**	Edit
BEATS PER MINUTE	
49 - 127	Nov 24, 2016 ⟩
44 - 138	Nov 23, 2016 ⟩
51 - 94	Nov 22, 2016 ⟩
46 - 90	Nov 21, 2016 ⟩

8 Tap on a day's results to view the times at which individual readings were taken

⟨ Back **All Recorded Data**	Edit
BEATS PER MINUTE	
🕐 66	Nov 24, 16:57 ⟩
🕐 65	Nov 24, 16:49 ⟩
🕐 67	Nov 24, 16:45 ⟩
🕐 59	Nov 24, 16:40 ⟩

Hot tip

Viewing individual segments of heart rate data is a good way to see the difference between your heart rate when doing exercise and at rest.

170

9 Tap on a specific heart rate item to view its details, such as time of recording and source device for recording

⟨ All Recorded Data **Details**
SAMPLE DETAILS
Heart Rate
66 bpm
Date
Nov 24, 2016, 16:57:14
Source
Nick's Apple Watch
Date Added to Health
Nov 24, 2016, 16:58:49
DEVICE DETAILS
Name
Apple Watch

Wireless Monitors

The sensors on the Apple Watch only monitor heart rate, but there is a range of wireless devices that can, in conjunction with the Apple Watch and iPhone, be used to monitor a more extensive range of health vitals, including blood pressure, weight management, and heart health. This requires the following:

- The appropriate wireless device. This is usually fitted around the arm, from where it measures the required health vitals.

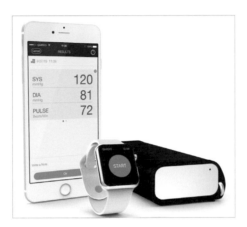

Beware

When looking for wireless health monitors, make sure that they are compatible with the iPhone and the Apple Watch.

- A companion app on the Apple Watch or iPhone, which collects the data from the wireless device.

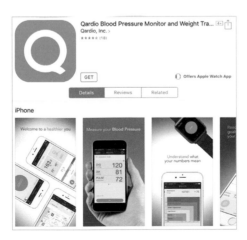

Hot tip

In some locations, health data from wireless monitors can be shared directly with doctors. This is mainly in some American states, but it is likely to be an area that expands in the future.

- The device has to be paired with the Apple Watch and the iPhone, using the **Bluetooth** setting.

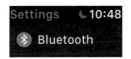

Tracking Diet

A healthy diet is an important part of overall health and fitness, but with all of the demands of modern life, it can sometimes be hard to maintain a healthy diet. To help with this, there are numerous apps that can be used to encourage a healthy diet and keep a record of what you eat and drink. These can be found in the App Store, and a lot of diet tracking apps have versions for the Apple Watch and the iPhone. To find these:

Don't forget

Accessing the App Store from the Watch app ensures that the apps that are displayed are compatible with the Apple Watch. If you only want to use them on the iPhone, access them from the App Store app on your iPhone.

172

1 Tap on the **Watch** app on the iPhone Home screen

Watch

2 Tap on the **Search** button on the bottom toolbar to open the App Store at the search page

Search

3 Enter **Diet Tracker** as the search keywords (or just **Diet**) and tap on the **Search** button, or tap on one of the search suggestions

diet tracker
calorie counter & diet tracker by myfitnesspal
calorie counter and diet tracker on 2016
low carb diet tracker pro by carb manager
mango - calories counter & diet tracker

Search

4 Swipe down the page to view all of the available diet trackers (these can be used on the iPhone and the Apple Watch. They can also be used solely on the iPhone, if required)

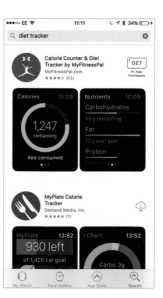

5 Tap on a diet tracker app to view its details. Tap on the **Get** button (or price button if it is a paid-for app) to download it

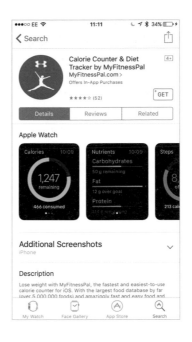

Using a diet tracker

Diet tracker apps mostly operate in a similar way, by calculating the number of calories consumed by the user against the amount of exercise, to provide a figure for the number of calories burned (or gained) and equating this into a weight loss figure. To use a diet tracker app (illustrated here with MyPlate):

For most diet tracker apps, you have to register with them using an email address and password before you can start using the app.

1 When the app is first accessed, you will be asked to enter some details including, age, gender, height, weight and goal, e.g. weight loss, and a target

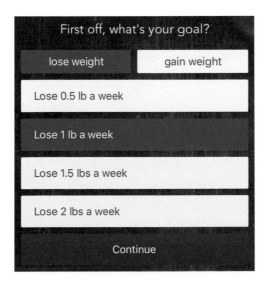

173

...cont'd

Don't forget

Diet trackers display a daily calorie goal, which is calorie intake minus the amount of exercise: the daily figure is the one calculated to achieve your desired weight.

Hot tip

When entering items you have eaten, you can enter a word in the search box and various matching options will be available. Tap on one of these, or items can be added manually.

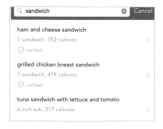

Some apps, like MyPlate, can scan types of food from their barcode. Tap on the Scan button and use the camera on the iPhone to scan the item.

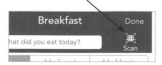

2 A lot of diet tracker apps request permission to access the Health app on your iPhone so that it can share information with it. Drag the buttons to **On** for the items of information that you want to share and tap on the **Allow** button

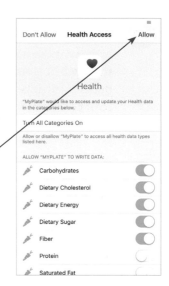

3 Diet tracker apps require you to list what you eat for each meal, which is used to calculate your calorie intake, and is then offset against the number of calories burned through exercise. Tap on a meal heading, e.g. breakfast

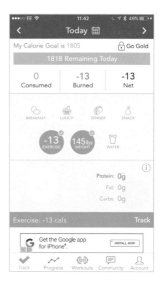

4 Enter what you ate for the selected meal. This can be done by entering the details in the search box, selecting items from a pre-populated list or, for some apps, scanning the item of food itself. Tap on the **Done** button once you have added the required item(s)

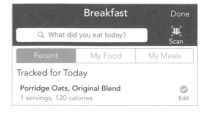

5 The meal details are displayed, including the amount of the serving, the date recorded, and the total number of calories consumed for the meal

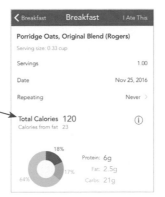

6 Each meal that is recorded is given a figure for the number of calories consumed

7 Details for exercise and weight are also available (the exercise figure is recorded from the Apple Watch or the iPhone)

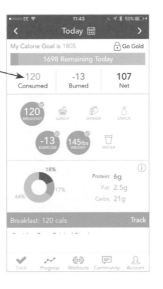

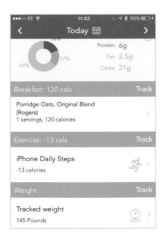

Beware

Dietary details cannot usually be entered on the app on the Apple Watch; it has to be done on the iPhone, and the details can then be viewed on the Apple Watch.

8 The information from the app is replicated on the Apple Watch version

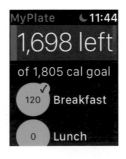

Healthy Eating

One of the keys to maintaining health and fitness (and achieving weight loss, if desired) is eating healthily. This does not mean that you have to eat healthy food all of the time, with no treats, but it is a good habit to get into as part of a long-term goal of improving your health and fitness. Some areas of healthy eating and diet to consider are:

Hot tip

One of the best reasons to cook your own food using fresh produce is that it generally tastes a lot better than ready meals or pre-packaged food. Also, you can make it to exactly your own tastes.

- **Eat as much fresh produce as possible**. Try to avoid ready meals and pre-packaged food, as it is harder to know what is actually in them.

- **Cook food from scratch**. Cooking your own food is an excellent way to see exactly what is being used. It does not have to be a long, time-consuming process, and lots of healthy and tasty meals can be cooked in the time it takes to go and buy a ready meal.

- **Try new recipes**. If you feel like you are getting fed up with the same meals, try something new. This will not only expand your cooking repertoire, but also add some variety into your healthy eating plan.

- **Use smaller plates**. If you are looking to cut down on the amount you eat, try using slightly smaller plates, which should lead to smaller portion sizes.

- **Don't restrict yourself too much**. Healthy eating should not be seen as a chore, and you should still allow yourself treats: the key is moderation.

- **If you are looking to lose weight, think of it as a long-term plan, rather than a quick fix over a few weeks**. Don't be too concerned about weighing yourself every day, but rather concentrate on how you feel in yourself. Look at it as a change in lifestyle instead of a fixed-term diet, and do not put pressure on yourself to see immediate results.

- **Look for encouragement for your healthy eating regime**. This does not have to be an organized club or diet-plan: family and friends are probably the best-placed people to share ideas, recipes and experiences with, and if it is seen as more of a communal activity it will provide long-term benefits for a greater number of people.

Healthy eating apps

Healthy eating and recipe apps can be downloaded from the App Store and used on the Apple Watch and iPhone. To do this:

1 Tap on the **Watch** app on the iPhone Home screen

2 Tap on the **Search** button on the bottom toolbar to open the App Store at the search page

3 Enter **Healthy eating** as the search keywords (or **Healthy recipes**) and tap on the **Search** button, or tap on one of the search suggestions

4 The healthy eating apps cover a range of topics including healthy recipes, weight loss plans, and lifestyle choices such as veganism or vegetarianism

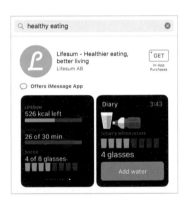

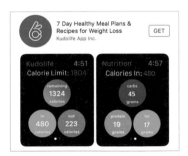

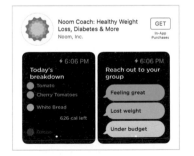

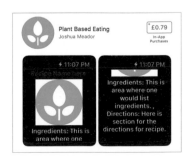

If you do not have an Apple Watch, the apps can be downloaded to your iPhone from the App Store app.

The apps illustrated in Step 4 are:

- **Lifesum**, which creates a plan from your lifestyle and healthy eating goals.

- **7 Day Healthy Meal Plans & Recipes for Weight Loss**, which suggests healthy meals to help you meet any weight loss goals you may have.

- **Noom Coach**, which also covers healthy eating, through the use of coached programs and also touches on preventing conditions such as Type 2 diabetes.

- **Plant Based Eating**, which covers vegetarian diet and the benefits that it can confer.

Sleep

Getting a good night's sleep is an important, and sometimes overlooked, aspect of overall health and fitness. Length and quality of sleep are both important, and there are some apps that can be used to help monitor your sleep patterns:

Hot tip

The App Store contains a range of apps for monitoring babies' sleep and feeding times.

178

1 Tap on the **Watch** app on the iPhone Home screen

2 Tap on the **Search** button on the bottom toolbar to open the App Store at the search page

3 Enter **Sleep** as the search keyword, and tap on one of the results

4 Sleep apps can monitor your sleep, including periods of deep sleep, and provide relaxing sounds to help you get to sleep. The iPhone or Apple Watch has to be located near to you when you are sleeping so that the app can monitor your sleeping from your breathing

Don't forget

The apps illustrated in Step 4 are:

- **Pillow**, which is a sleep tracker for measuring the length and quality of your sleep.

- **Sleep++**, another sleep tracker.

- **TaoMix**, which can be used to help you get to sleep through a range of soothing sounds.

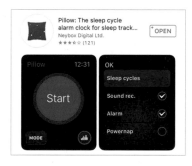

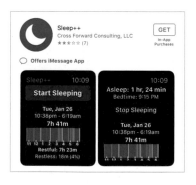

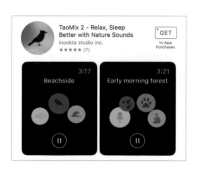

Mindfulness

Mindfulness is another term for relaxation, covering areas such as meditation, sleep and general relaxation. The Health app on the iPhone has a category for entering mindfulness, and there is also a range of apps in the App Store that can be used on the iPhone and the Apple Watch for relaxation:

1 Tap on the **Watch** app on the iPhone Home screen

2 Tap on the **Search** button on the bottom toolbar to open the App Store at the search page

3 Enter **Mindfulness** as the search keyword, and tap on one of the results

4 The majority of mindfulness apps cover meditation, but there are also some apps that cover brain training for mindfulness, breathing techniques, and sleep

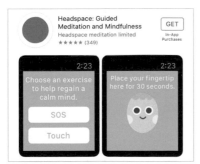

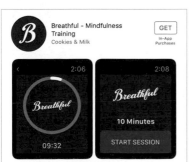

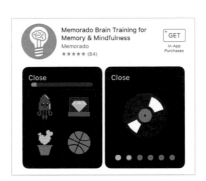

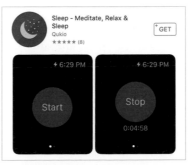

The Breathe app on the Apple Watch can also be used to remind you to pause and take some deep breaths for a few minutes for relaxation during the day.

The apps illustrated in Step 4 are:

- **Headspace**, which offers guided meditation for all ages.

- **Memorado Brain Training for Memory & Mindfulness**, which offers a brain training program that can be used to aid meditation and relaxation.

- **Breathful**, which offers meditation sessions and also tracks their effectiveness.

- **Sleep – Meditate, Relax & Sleep**, which can be used for more relaxing sleep patterns.

Health and Fitness Equipment

Having good equipment is important for any sporting activity, and this is certainly true for health and fitness. This helps you in a range of activities, and buying new equipment can give you a boost in terms of enthusiasm and motivation.

Footwear

Good footwear is probably the most important item in terms of health and fitness activities. Whether it is for running or walking, or for doing general workouts, a good quality pair of shoes will aid in terms of the activity itself and also help protect your joints from the impact of the activity.

Breathable clothing

Proper sports clothing helps you feel better about yourself when you are exercising, and also ensures that you feel as fresh as possible. Look for items that are breathable, i.e. ones that remove sweat away from the body and help you stay as cool as possible.

Water bottles

Drinking plenty of water is important during any sporting activity, so using a water bottle should always be considered essential.

Exercise balls

Large rubber balls are used in activities such as Pilates and are useful for general workouts, particularly for improving stomach muscles and general flexibility.

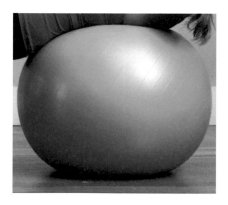

Exercise mats

For activities such as yoga, an exercise mat is important for doing work on the floor, and also for workout exercises that require you to lie on the floor, such as for sit-ups.

Weights

If you want to do strengthening work, a set of weights is a good option. This can be in the form of hand-held dumbbells, or larger weights for activities such as bench-pressing.

Hot tip

Try to buy the best pair of shoes that you can, as they will serve you well in terms of performance and protection.

Hot tip

For runners and walkers, small backpack water carriers are an excellent option. They are relatively small and lightweight, and have a tube that is used for drinking while you are running or walking.

10 Creating a Health and Fitness Regime

This chapter looks at some long-term ways to maintain health and fitness.

Motivation

Embracing a comprehensive health and fitness regime is something that should stand you in good stead for your whole life. However, it is something that can be time-consuming and hard to maintain over a long period of time. Being motivated, and staying motivated, are important factors when looking to create a long-term health and fitness regime. Some areas to consider are:

- **You have to want to do it**. The most important type of motivation is within yourself, and from a genuine desire to undertake a new health and fitness lifestyle. If you are half-hearted, or reluctant to start with, then you are probably destined to fail.

- **Establish a routine**. Health and fitness should be considered a normal part of your day/week. In order to embed this with your other activities, create a routine for your health and fitness, e.g. going for a run on certain days each week, or going for a walk every lunchtime at work. It should become second-nature, rather than something that is considered out of the ordinary.

- **Don't be afraid to change your routine**. Even when you have established a regular routine, it can be beneficial to change it from time to time, just so that you do not become bored with your activities. This can be doing them at a different time and day, or changing the type of activity so that you do something different now and again.

Beware

If you give yourself rewards in the form of your favorite food or drink, do not overdo it otherwise this could negate the good work done through the physical activity.

- **Using rewards**. Giving yourself virtual and actual rewards is another way to keep motivated. Apps such as the Activity app on the iPhone and the Apple Watch have a range of awards that you can acquire, and this is a surprisingly effective way to make you want to reach your goals. Awards can be achieved for individual workouts or for succeeding in meeting targets over a period of time. In addition, give yourself some actual rewards as well as the virtual ones.

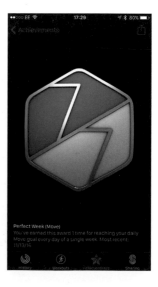

- **Buy new equipment**. One way to maintain motivation is to buy new equipment: if you have a new pair of shoes or clothing you will probably feel more inclined to perform some exercise just so that you can use them.

- **Collaborate with others**. Getting encouragement from other people is an excellent way to keep motivated, whether this is by sharing health and fitness details virtually or by engaging in activities with other people so that you can encourage each other, and exercising becomes more of a communal activity. Items can be shared from the Activity app by tapping on the Share button. The method of sharing is then selected, e.g. Messages, Mail or social media.

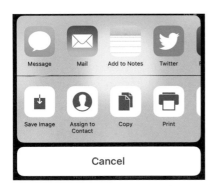

The relevant item is added to the selected app for sharing. This can be your daily activity rings for different types of activity...

...or details of any virtual awards that you have received.

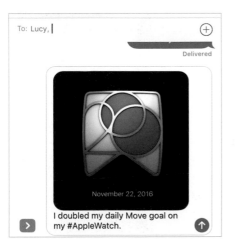

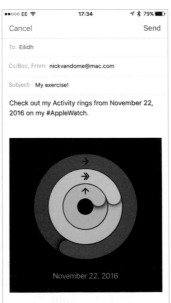

Beware

Do not bombard people with details of your fitness activities, as they may tire of it if you send them too many updates.

183

Being Realistic

One important aspect of health and fitness is to be realistic in terms of what you want to achieve and how quickly this can be done: achievable expectations are a lot better than hoping that you can be turned into an elite athlete overnight. Some things to consider when viewing your health and fitness activities are:

- Whatever your goals are, don't expect to reach them overnight. In sporting terms, look at it as a marathon rather than a sprint.

- Don't expect to see immediate result in terms of your appearance, e.g. if you want to get fitter and also achieve a level of weight loss.

- Don't make extravagant claims to other people about what you are going to achieve: this will only put more pressure on yourself and you may end up disappointed and unmotivated if you do not achieve what you hoped.

- Don't overdo it at the beginning. When you first start a new health and fitness regime it can be tempting to do as much as possible to begin with, as if this will store up fitness for the future. However, it could have a detrimental effect on your body and your muscles, as they may not be used to doing such a level of exercise. It is much better to build up slowly over a longer period of time.

- Understanding and accepting your own limitations. We generally know what our bodies can and cannot do, and it is important to recognize this. Also, as we get older it is not always possible to do the same levels of exercise as when we were younger, so this should be accepted too.

- Don't try to emulate what you see elite sportspeople doing. They are at the top of their profession for a reason, and undertake an awful lot of physical work that is not always seen or appreciated. Trying to do the same things could lead to injuries of varying degrees.

- Do expect that you will be able to start and maintain a health and fitness regime that can last a lifetime. There is no reason why this cannot be done by anyone, so it is important to realize this and plan your future exercise activities accordingly.

Hot tip

'Little and often' is a good approach to long-term health and fitness. Even short periods of physical activity can be beneficial, particularly if you do it frequently.

Setting Goals

One consideration when starting a new health and fitness regime is deciding what it is you want to get out of it. This can be in terms of short-term goals and also long-term ones.

Short-term goals

Some of the short-term goals to consider are:

- Establish health and fitness as part of your day-to-day activity. If you aim to have this embedded in your daily routine then it will quickly become second-nature.

- Ensure family and friends recognize your commitment to your health and fitness goals. If other people accept that this is part of your life, then it will be easier to maintain it.

- Make incremental improvements to the amount of exercise that you do. Try to make small increases to your activity, so that you have something to aim for each time you are exercising or performing a workout. They do not have to be significant increases (in fact, it is better to always work up in small amounts, but also consolidate at each new level).

- Competing with family and friends. Some friendly competition with like-minded people is a good way to make exercising more interesting: if someone is running or walking further than you, or doing longer workouts, set a goal of trying to match them, or surpass them. However, do this over a period of time rather than trying to do it too quickly.

Long-term goals

Some of the long-term goals to consider:

- Improve your overall health. This can be in terms of areas such as blood pressure or cholesterol levels. These can be compared if you have a general medical check-up at regular intervals, e.g. a yearly check-up.

- Lose weight. Not everyone wants to lose weight as a result fitness activities, but it is a common goal for many people. However, if this is something that you want to do, look at it over the long-term rather than a quick fix over a short period of time.

- Look to establish health and fitness as a lifelong activity.

Consult your own doctor for medical advice about how you can best improve your overall health and fitness.

Using Timescales

If health and fitness activities are viewed as a lifelong ambition, it can be useful to set timescale goals along the way:

Daily

Daily targets can be set for achieving specific goals, such as the three activity rings on the Activity app for the iPhone and Apple Watch. These are pre-set goals (apart from the Move goal, which is editable), and are achievable on a daily basis. Other health and fitness apps have similar daily targets: aiming to achieve these each day should be the initial target.

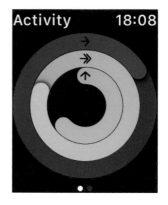

Weekly

Each week, try to add to the daily targets, or increase the targets themselves. Regardless of this, it is important to ensure that you meet your goals on a weekly basis, not just a daily one.

Monthly

As you progress with your health and fitness activities, a useful monthly goal is to try to achieve as many consecutive days of exercise as possible. Some apps provide rewards for consecutive days of activity, and this can be a good way to motivate yourself to keep going over a longer period of time.

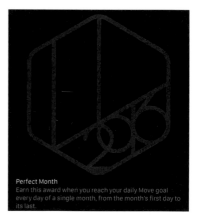

Perfect Month
Earn this award when you reach your daily Move goal every day of a single month, from the month's first day to its last.

Yearly

A yearly timescale can be set for an overall assessment of your health and fitness activities. You can look at what you have achieved in that time (make sure that you reward yourself for your efforts), and also set new goals and aims for the next year. Maintaining health and fitness should be looked at as a lifelong activity, and you should always be looking at how you can consolidate and improve on what you have been doing.

Index